Pangasm

Introducing the Feminine
Principle of Darkness

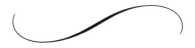

Lori S. Dante

iUniverse, Inc.
Bloomington

Pangasm
Introducing the Feminine Principle of Darkness

iUniverse books may be ordered through booksellers or by contacting:

iUniverse
1663 Liberty Drive
Bloomington, IN 47403
www.iuniverse.com
1-800-Authors (1-800-288-4677)

Cover Art by
Michael Abbey

ISBN: 978-1-4502-9790-5 (pbk)
ISBN: 978-1-4502-9792-9 (cloth)
ISBN: 978-1-4502-9791-2 (ebk)

Printed in the United States of America

iUniverse rev. date: 3/22/11

When I first decided to write a book detailing this principle in 2003, the world was in a very dark and foreboding place. In this environment I found constant support and love from Richard – the Lion Heart. His kindness and bravery are unmatched! And, dear Miss Rebecca spun light bridges across chasms of confusion every time I trusted myself to her attentive ministrations. And, the very warmth of life itself rests within the hearts of my children, to them I am home -- what more could a soul desire?

Pangasm is dedicated to the loving memory of my little brother Gib and to my dear mother for surviving such a terrible loss, while continuing to give of her caring love to one and all. Thank you.

A PORTION OF THE PROCEEDS FROM THE SALE OF THIS BOOK WILL BE DONATED TO A WATERSHED RECLAMATION PROJECT CALLED:

MAUKA MAKAI MAUI TRAILS or mmmtrails@msn.com

Contents

Introduction

Ahhh! The "Love Cocktail", made from our own body and stimulated by sexual excitement. This elixir is comprised of dopamine, fenylethylamine, adrenaline, endorphins, vasopressin and oxytocin, and is a cocktail of yumminess that floods our bloodstream helping us to feel heaven on earth! This ecstatic formula is what scientists, the world over, have attempted to re-create to no avail. Even so, the Love Cocktail is available to anyone at any time, yet, has been lost to the collective misunderstanding about our human birthright and the glorious role that human emotion has in creating our reality. As a result of this misunderstanding, our sexual relations have become complicated and illusive, leaving many to believe that the word "relationship" is more like a four letter curse word!

I first considered writing Pangasm because my daughter was attempting to explain to her girlfriends the sexual concepts that I had been teaching her. Primarily, she was trying to describe "Spiritual Birth-Control" methods that we, and others, had been having success with. It was, and to some degree, still is, a major challenge to take what I had been studying for the past four decades and put it into a language that young adults could comprehend, especially since many scholars had trouble comprehending the Principle of Pangasm. Now, almost eight years later, I am still attempting to get the language "right". As many of you may already know, the abstinence program adopted by the US government to combat teen pregnancy has not changed the ongoing problem of un-planned pregnancy. It is my hope that we can alter this unfortunate pattern with education, rather than blame and shame that does not help anyone.

My only qualification for writing a book about human sexuality is that I am a sexual woman, a mother and a grandmother. When asked to qualify my expertise, I had to ask myself "what is an expert?" Many people consider expertise as a result of education, but let's not forget that true expertise comes from experience. Most mothers have a genuine expertise that comes from an all-encompassing desire to create a safe environment for their children. I taught my children the core spiritual aspects of Free Will and how this relates to our sexual pro-creative attributes. The core aspect of the *Principle of Pangasm* is the actualization of PERSONAL SOVEREIGNTY (Free Will) as it relates to developing our own lifestyle and our own ability to pro-create or not pro-create children. I have come to realize that the term Personal Sovereignty is a very broad term that means many things to many people. Suffice it to say that this principle leads us into a greater awareness of the unique truth that each of us harbors as PERSONALITY. Simply educating ourselves about the fundamental electro-magnetic nature of our human personality empowers us to create a life that continually supports our Will to live, if we so desire.

Each of us have unique problems that require unique solutions -- in this spirit I wish to qualify that each and every one of us is an expert about our own individual truth. The Principle of Pangasm is designed to help you locate these solutions without becoming subject to the truth of others. To the extent that this truth aligns with the LAWS OF NATURE will be the extent to which any individual will enjoy success in making their dreams come true. I have done my best to describe these laws in simple terms so that you can work within these limits to devise custom-made practical applications that thrill your heart.

I re-wrote this book 5 times in an attempt to get close to the language that would help anyone to better understand their sexual birthright. Why? Originally, I thought this work was about Spiritual Birth-control, but, when I approached a certain segment of our society to proclaim the good news of our positive results, I was demonized and even received death threats! As a result, I came to the realization that the misunderstandings about human sexuality have led our confused populace into dark alleyways of contempt and violence! I was terrified for my children and I, as a result, I changed the book to exclude any mention of *Spiritual Birth Control* methods. I have since resolved my fear and have evolved a well-grounded understanding of survival terror as it relates to this principle, and in a way that I am now privileged to offer. This was no small feat! Originally, the terror that arose from receiving death threats converted to anger and righteous indignation, then converted to rage and paranoia; but, I did not wish to make this book about that, instead, I chose to write a book outlining a principle that explains the Laws of Nature in electromagnetic terms, but also as a way of taking the charge (blame and shame) out of the diverse personal opinions about the current state of the Human Condition that is the *Battle of the Sexes*.

Originally, I called this book "*Dieting, Dating and Death – The Three D's of Devolution*". Even though that title describes the symptoms of the *Battle of the Sexes*, it was more about the problem than it was about the solution. This edition of *Pangasm* will not delve into spiritual birth-control issues, simply because I feel that it confuses the primary issue, which is: How does one practically apply the *Principle of Pangasm* to their sexual relationships and to their mental, emotional and physical health. This is such a broad topic that covers all aspects of life, that rushing in to heap on controversial issues (such as birth-control) could only serve to confound the student of Pangasm.

I cannot lead you in the ways in which I have chosen to create personal balance, since balance for me may not fit your dream of what balance means for you. Whether it is better health, greater intimacy, improved living situations, more freedom or more excitement, our individual desire is unique and any pre-conceived notions by me, or anyone else calling themselves an expert, should not be put forward as a custom-made solution for you. Therefore, I have done my best to detail the *Principle of Pangasm* as insight into the electromagnetic aspect of personality and free Will in such a way that you will be inspired to envision the future to suit your unique heart's desire and wholeheartedly open to your own creative ability to do so.

I was raised in the 1950's where young men and women were caught between the traditional sexual norms and the new age of sexual openness that was culminating in the 1960's through the "Flower Children" or "Hippy" movement. Within this context, I found myself spiritually bankrupt at an early age! Therefore, I have spent my entire life studying human sexuality to find solutions for myself and for my family. As a mother, I felt a deep need to discuss this with my children in the same spirit of openness of my generation, but I did not wish to poison them with guilt or condemn their sexual explorations as being wrong simply because I had now come to a place of understanding about the actual bio-spiritual ramifications of human orgasm, which I have formulated as the *Principle of Pangasm*.

I found the sexual ethic that evolved from my generation, and down into my children's generation, to be dark and particularly abusive toward women; given that my generation ushered in "Women's Liberation" it seemed unfortunate that there was such a backlash for women from this social experiment. This is not what my generation was attempting to create, but the backlash against sexual openness was and is a violent, shaming rage for good reason -- sexuality that is shared in the presence of denied self-hatred and guilt creates hell on earth. I know this may sound rather radical, but the results of sharing sexual orgasm in the presence of guilt can create any number of ungrounded and deadly scenarios that play themselves out in the news on a daily basis. I so wanted my children to experience the beauty, joy and love that comes from sex in the presence of openness and self-love, rather than the current "gangsta-style" dehumanization of sex being depicted in popular culture. This is one of the many reasons why I created the *GAME OF PANGASM* -- to counter the dark emptiness of gangsta sex that is absent of romantic magic.

My challenge is to help those who play this game to be able to utilize it for its intended therapeutic purpose, rather than take this amazing game out of context and possibly confuse the participants further. The first 5 chapters of this book describe the Principle in elemental terms to help the reader further understand the power of personality as described in chapter 6. As a result of understanding and aligning our personality with the Laws of Nature, the reader will more than likely wish to share this blessing with others, especially when it comes to playing the game with people we are sexually attracted to! When we comprehend the metaphysical patterns that the physical realm stems from, then we can begin to evolve deeper understandings by playing the game and stimulating our energetic matrix to become reciprocal.

The *Principle of Pangasm* is based upon energetic patterns that have been measured by modern science and verified by biological patterns that constitute "The Laws of Nature." The 5 elements that comprise life on earth are: ***EARTH, FIRE, WATER, ETHER AND AIR.*** These primary elements are the building blocks of physical existence, and amazingly enough, they are responsive to personality. I will detail the ways in which dense physical matter is magical in an easy to understand language that will help any Harry Potter fan to realize that magic isn't just a fictional tale. The stuff that constitutes the realm of Time and Space is an evolving perfection that has, within its design, the properties of dense physical matter that are responsive to personality. We have called this magical, miraculous and even the Devil's work, depending on our understanding of our human nature.

Ultimately, you are the only authority about your own truth and your decision-making process, as long as this truth aligns with the *Laws of Nature.* Choosing to live by your own unique truth, versus living according to the beliefs of others, is a powerful way to live and inspires our heart into the rewards of creativity and individuality. Unfortunately, many spiritual concepts see the human ego as the source of imbalance, whereas, I see the ego as being caught in a no-win game that is held present by a collective misunderstanding that rarely, if ever, gets questioned. It is important not to throw the ego out with the bathwater!

While reading Pangasm, some of you may experience temporary illness, confusion, strong emotions, etc....since the process is unique for each person, keep an open heart for a principle that is designed to lead us into ever-greater levels of health, self-awareness and freedom, regardless of our initial reaction to the information.

A common definition of the *'BATTLE OF THE SEXES'* describes a situation where two people want to do two different things, but do them together. This accurately describes the electromagnetic conundrum that energetically creates this unfortunate and repetitive scenario. By studying the basic energetic patterns of electromagnetism, we develop understandings of the nature of human magnetism and how it is we constantly create intimidating form, rather than the stuff of our dreams.

Fortunately, one of the benefits of being human is that we do not need others in order to utilize the miraculous healing power of orgasmic sexual ether. Having said that, orgasm that is experienced within the current belief structure (paradigm) of mankind is somewhat like being bludgeoned to death with joy! Because, we have been using one of the most blessed gifts in creation to create the ongoing *Battle of the Sexes*!

NOTE: Pangasm is a highly sexual game -- albeit a technically non-sexual encounter -- that helps the players get attuned with the presence of sexual ether, without engaging in sexual intercourse or oral sex. In this way, it is possible to share heightened levels of sexual excitement that heals, without plunging the players into any residual remorse, shame or negative physical repercussions. The primary physical repercussions that come from playing this game are physical, mental, emotional and spiritual rejuvenation, as well as, enabling a sexual pair to experience the beauty of intimacy shared within the spirit of Personal Sovereignty.

CHAPTER ONE

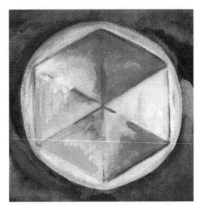

ELEMENT EARTH

GAIA

The word *Pangasm* is the word used to describe the force and influence of mankind's collective orgasmic energy. *"Pan"* is Latin meaning *"All"*, and *"gasm"* is a derivative of the word *"orgasm"*. Humanity enjoys bio-spiritual attributes that have been known about for eons and there is vast information in the way of spiritual, and/or magical, abilities that have been handed down since the beginning of history. Today, we are discovering evidence that the earth has been the home of ancient civilizations that had superior knowledge of astronomy, alchemy and possibly extra-terrestrial travel, as well, an intimate awareness of human energetic systems. But, very little has been offered in the way of understanding the role of human emotions regarding the fantastic birthright that bio-spiritual personality has available to it. The *Principle of Pangasm* is a concept (based in science and founded upon the romantic nature of electromagnetism) detailing the components of personality and how they operate; outlining dynamic means of aligning these parts of self with the *Laws of Nature* and thereby enabling the reader to resolve the age old *Battle of the Sexes* within their own self. By simply understanding this principle, one opens the way for *Providence* to support and lead a person into the ways of enjoying the fruits of True Free Will.

Here we are on Earth, spinning through Dark Matter on a carbon ball of life following patterns set into motion 13.5 billion years ago when our Universe emerged from the Big Bang of expansion. Even though science has mapped the human genome, it has failed to measure the Romantic Nature of the Sun and the Earth as being the two most biologically influential beings in our daily life. We do not relate to their gravity as Love or their electromagnetic connection as romantic in nature, but consider for a moment, that the Laws of Nature are bio-spiritually romantic? In accordance with the *Principle of Pangasm*, Gaia (the Earth) has a lover who is the center of her Universe and whom the ancient Greeks referred to as Helios. She is his Yin (darkness) and he is her Yang (light).

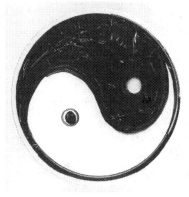

'YINYANG'

She is the dark liquid heart that he shines his never-failing, ever-constant light into. His are the macrocosmic arms of the paternal source of fire, ever-holding her close in his embrace. She is the warm breast that suckles our every need; and, we are a Star's way of seeing itself. The electromagnetic matrix of a human being follows closely that of our Solar System. The Earth is our root that magnetically binds us to our great matriarch. The sun is our crown and the great patriarch of the heavens providing us with the Direct Current (DC) of the element of fire. We each have this microcosmic root (our body) and this crown (our brain). The root is the magnetic dark aspect, or negative polarity of density, and the crown is the electric aspect or positive polarity of light.

If our birthright is an energetic equilibrium that sustains perfect health, why has mankind not enjoyed such a fate until now? Because an ancient misunderstanding has rendered the matrix of our Light Body to systematically repel the electric from the magnetic within each individual at an early age. This is collectively demonstrated by a split mind, violence, neglect and despair called *THE BATTLE OF THE SEXES*. This problem makes the electric part of us stop exchanging properties with the magnetic part of us, essentially leading individuals and the collective to produce chronic imbalance that we have called "normal."

In the case of simple magnets, we can see two magnets that are polarized to positive and negative holding one another together as a result of an invisible and silent energetic bond. Likewise, when two magnets are polarized to the same polarity, as in positive/positive or negative/negative, we then see the two magnets repel away from each other with this same force. When humans polarize in this way, they are energetically mimicking the Battle of the Sexes. Even though we cannot see, hear or smell this energy, it is nonetheless real; essentially, energy is the foundation and source of complex organisms like our selves.

The Greek philosopher Paracleseus (1493 to 1541) described the phenomenon of Chi (referred to here as the element Ether): "The vital force is not enclosed in man, but radiates around him like a luminous sphere, and it may be made to act at a distance. In these semi-material rays, the imagination of a man may produce health or morbidity". Thus, it has been known down through the ages, that the life force of Chi is the foundation for being physical.

3

The *Principle of Pangasm* classifies the elemental-environment into 5 major groupings: **EARTH, FIRE, WATER, AIR and ETHER;** and, classifies the 4 parts of personality as the familial archetypes of: **Father, Mother, Son and Daughter** to symbolize the parts of personality that must align with the elemental world. When considering the parts of personality, it can be helpful to also view them as the four directions: **North/electric, South/magnetic, East/heart and West/body.** These cognitive connections will help us identify with the disparate parts of self that have been stuck in an electromagnetic conundrum that we have collectively chosen to perceive as normal and/or inevitable. Through relating to the parts of this battle as vital aspects that need to align with life and by understanding the nature of the elements of density, the way opens for the personality to identify opportunities and possibilities that were not previously understood as available.

The LAWS OF NATURE provide the ELEMENTS that are responsive to personality, and through aligning our parts of personality with life -- we are then given the capacity to establish Personal Sovereignty, which is true Free Will. Our birthright is a glorious foundation that many would call magical and the truth is that self-love and insight into the Laws of Nature can lead us into creating a life that is free from over-control, violence, disparity and debility. The process of aligning our personality can be as confusing and frightening as the current confusing and frightening scenarios of the human condition. Having said that, I am here to report that the results of this effort have, and remain, fascinating and rewarding.

When it comes to aligning the *FOUR PARTS OF PERSONALITY*, understanding what these parts are and how they function is the solution to resolving the current Human Condition that is steeped in the *Battle of the Sexes*. Due to a mass hypnosis that happens to one and all, regardless of where one lives or what language one speaks, our electromagnetic mechanism polarizes into two separate entities that no longer reciprocate electric essence (Silver Chi) with the magnetic essence (Golden Chi) in our heart. As a result of this indoctrination process, human beings begin the aging process at an early age. It has been next to impossible to identify this collective problem due to the collective paradigm (the belief structure of mankind) that is considered as: all there is to reality.

The Four Parts of Personality need to align as one perspective. Consider that North, South, East and West are identifiable as the archetypes of family: Father (North=Electric Brain); Mother (South=magnetic emotions) and East and West represent the Twin Hearts (Son/body and Daughter/heart) that conduct the magic of North and South in our heart and through the left and right hands. When our heart conducts the electric Chi with the magnetic Chi, our hands and, indeed, our entire body conducts the healing energy of self-love that is capable of loving the other; this is the pathway into the sublime realm of un-conditional love. Consider for a moment the veritable impossibility of experiencing un-conditional love if one's own basic needs are not being met. The no-win situation of the *Battle of the Sexes* imposes just such a challenge upon the hearts of mankind. This is not the result of being "bad" it is simply a long-standing misunderstanding that has one and all looking for a "bad guy" to blame for what we have collectively created.

Without physical health, the mind begins to decline and so does our Will to live. The height of an aligned Personality is the ability to maintain physical health and vitality in a way that supports our Will to live. Therefore, un-locking the mysteries of dense physicality is one of my favorite pastimes. I find my body to be a universe of wonder and the more I learn about my cellular biology, the more my love for my human form develops in earnest. As a result of this awareness and appreciation, I have come to have intimate relation with my organs and I am fascinated with what is being revealed to me through this dynamic and intimate relationship with my form. Each of my organs has a voice that is unique and responsive. Often, when I refer to the miraculous nature of the human heart, my own heart skips a beat and gives me a flutter.

What constitutes the matter of density, such as that of our flesh-and-blood body and that of the earth itself? By relating to the elements that comprise dense form, dealing with the fundamental function of a human body can become less mysterious and intimidating. Our physical presence is part and parcel of the element Earth, comprising many properties in the same way that a human body is a universe unto itself. Today, we are witness to an epochal earth-changing Melt Water event. There are many factors influencing the earth's *Resonant Frequency* to rise significantly in modern times likewise, there is a correlation between the earth's rising frequency and the Melt Water that is currently escalating and causing a global conversation about the ramifications of Global Warming.[1]

Today, our earth is entering into a cycle that has been deemed a *"Star-Gate"* by many astronomers, as well as students of Metaphysical traditions. Many know this event as coined by students of the ancient Mayan Astronomy in relation to the Solstice of 2012. Interestingly enough, astronomical scientists have verified that there is an alignment occurring between our sun and the central sun of the Milky Way galaxy. I will describe this galactic process in later chapters and wish to point out that, as a race we are entering into a "QUICKENING" that is demonstrated by an escalating planetary frequency and a Melt Water event that is marked by melting glaciers and the North and South poles. Many believe that, this cycle has been made extreme because of increased CO_2 (carbon dioxide) emissions caused by the Industrial Age. As with any complex organism, the earth has many mechanisms that allow her to maintain atmospheric balance, much as a human body has the ability to regulate its vital organs into a well-functioning microcosm of the planet that gave birth to our race. According to the *Principle of Pangasm*, human evolution is closely related to the earth's predisposition toward her creation, mankind.

---

1   DEFINITITION FOR RESONANT FREQUENCY: All vibrating things in this world have their own, "natural" frequency, which they are most comfortable with. When a thing is subjected to an external force that makes it vibrate at a frequency it vibes with the most, the thing responds by vibrating at the maximum amplitude (energy). This phenomenon manifests throughout the universe. This natural frequency of that thing or body is known as its "resonating" or "resonant" frequency, and the phenomenon is known as "Resonance".

This dynamic relationship is highly intimate, and thanks to recent scientific discovery, it is possible to demonstrate this as a beautiful fact that is due to the *Laws of Nature*.

The emotional self is the source of our magnetic ether and is derived from the earth herself; however, emotions are deeply misunderstood today and *Pangasm* is designed to help us understand what energetic role human emotions play in maintaining electromagnetic balance or preventing it. In Chapter Four, the element ether is discussed at length as the *Genii in our Bottle*; this life-force plasma is also responsive to our belief-structure and is felt as human emotion. In essence, this ether is derived from the gravity of earth and is made unique by our signature resonant frequency as defined by our unique personality. Not only does our emotional nature constitute the magnetic aspect of our electromagnetic Light Body, it is also essential to the function of human magnetism because it is what draws our experiences to us.

In the past, humanity did not know what role human emotions played in creating our reality and only recently has it been discovered by NASA'S GOES SATELLITE observations that human emotions influence the strength and nature of earth's magnetic field, giving new meaning to the term: "As within, so it is without".

Gregg Braden's book "Fractal Time: Magnetic Fields and Life", discusses evidence discovered by GOES SATELLITES indicating that the earth's magnetic field not only affects the human psyche and physiology, likewise, heartfelt human emotion affect the earth's magnetic fields. These satellites made fascinating observations about the changes made to the earth's magnetic field during the events of 9/11: "From a location of about 22,300 miles above the equator, GOES 8 detected the first surge followed by an upward trend in the readings that topped out at nearly 50 units (Nano-Teslas) higher than any that had been typical for the same time previously. The time was 9:00 A.M. Eastern standard time; 15 minutes after the first plane hit the World Trade Center and about 15 minutes before the second impact."

"Subsequent studies by Princeton University and The Institute of HeartMath, (an innovative research institution formed in 1991 to pioneer research and development of heart-based technologies), have found that it appears to be the heart-based emotion of the world's population during such events that seems to be influencing the magnetic fields of the Earth! What makes this discovery so significant is that those fields are now linked to everything from the stability of the climate to the peace between nations." (*Fractal Time: Magnetic fields and Life*, by Gregg Braden

This is substantial evidence about our inter-connectedness with earth! The earth element, as it appears, is personified as Gaia and contains all the properties essential to our survival; in essence, the earth is the ultimate element, behaving as a loving mother suckling her 7-plus billion babies. If the earth responds to situations such as, the global outcry over the bombing of the World Trade Center, we can begin to recognize the amazing responsiveness that constitutes the *LAWS OF NATURE* that beautifully support Free Will for Personality.

The primary element that helps the earth meld plants, animals and people from her depths is cosmic dust, which is the very stuff of earth's mantel that is floating on the magma seas as Tectonic Plates. The tremendous discovery of Microzyma granules (cosmic dust particulates that form all plants, blood and tissue on earth) in 1866 by a French scientist named Antoine Bechamp, was a revolution of information that was largely ignored until recently. (*"SICK AND TIRED? Claim Your Inner Terrain"* by, DR. Robert O. Young and Shelly Redford Young: Woodland Publishing)

Microzyma means "small ferment," describing how these cosmic dust particles are triggers within our cells that are responsive to the pH environment of the cell. Through fermentation, the microzymian process produces continual cellular breakdown simultaneously with cellular renewal. Essentially, the *Microzymian Principle* is a biological model of electromagnetic cellular balance:

"IF THE ENVIRONMENT OF A CELL'S pH IS OUT OF BALANCE, THAT CELL WILL MUTATE ITSELF INTO THE SAME BACTERIA, FUNGI, YEAST, AND MOLD THAT FERMENT A DEAD BODY." Dr. Peter Young.

In other words, our cells can live in a state of reciprocal harmony with each other if they are in electromagnetic balance (a suitable pH) or the Microzyma can change our cells into a morbid state that eventually eliminates our existence. This is PLEOMORPHISM (as defined by Merriam-Webster dictionary as: "the quality or state of having or assuming various forms").

Pleomorphism is the constant variable of the Microzymian Principle that establishes cellular adaptation, known as evolution.

Just as Gaia maintains a resonant frequency that is her astronomical signature, a human Light Body determines our physical disposition by maintaining a resonant frequency capable of supporting cellular renewal. It is important to understand that the Light Body springs from the consciousness of personality and not the other way around. As to whether or not the Light Body is capable of reciprocity between its negative and positive poles, this is determined by the individual self-concept or paradigm. Likewise, electromagnetic imbalance (constant stress creates depression = low resonant frequency) is a signal to nature to transform the organism that is suffering.

Interestingly enough, according to Bechamp's studies, our body naturally has the factors and potential necessary to produce the symptoms of disease without any outer contagions. Equally, humans have all the tools in their bodies to heal any malady, even the ugliness that comes from aging. The crucial thing to understand is that viruses, bacteria and fungi can evolve out of any cell in our body without contagious contact with the outside world. These agents of decomposition are the result of microzyma responding to a chronically acidic pH, which is caused by stress and/or improper nutrition and/or lack of movement (low vibration). Either way, this ultimately stems from what it is the personality believes and, therefore, does.

One of the fascinating aspects of Bechamp's research is the fact that microzyma never die! Even after the body that was the host of the microzyma is decomposed after death. The microzyma (which is simply responsive cosmic dust) lives on. This is a biological fact that takes us into a realm that is seemingly magic. However, most people have an acidic pH leading to a host of symptoms that I would need another book to describe. Modern medicine is just now waking up to the vital affect that pH has upon our health, and eventually, most disorders will be treated by restoring the body's pH balance and improving all processes of elimination and renewal. However, if stress is not also addressed, then proper nutrition is hardly effective in counteracting the ravages of stress that cause our bodies to become acidic.

The earth is not necessarily a hostile hostess for she has held open her arms of unlimited abundance for evolutionary beings to evolve within, seemingly forever. The consciousness of unconditional love that emits from all plants in the form of oxygen and sustenance is her ever-present blessing. Gaia and Helios hold our North (positive) and South (negative) poles of existence faithfully, forever and a day, giving us life to share with one another. The Microzyma dust particles that comprise all blood, tissue and plant fiber are the building blocks of evolution and have guided our biological evolution since before time immemorial to this present moment where it is entirely possible to utilize this beautiful scientific fact to create and maintain perfect health.

Attending to the stress of unremitting survival terror is an aspect of modern society that is still largely misunderstood. The *Principle of Pangasm* is an introduction to the role that emotion plays in creating our health or causing our demise. For it is the emotional aspect of our nature that provides our magnetic movement, without magnetic presence and motion, the parts of personality begin to fall apart, much as our highly sophisticated societies fall apart with regularity.

Since our body is subject to our individual and collective paradigm, it is not possible to create lasting health without attending to the electrical thought-forms of *BELIEF*, as well as, the emotional disturbance that arises from the stress of having had adopted belief's that were founded upon misunderstanding. However, even erroneous belief's are capable of creating erroneous realities, likewise, belief's that are constructed within the context of the *Laws of Nature* have a powerful way of prevailing over the erroneous concepts... eventually.

Understanding the order of dense physicality can also be stated as "Bio-Centrism" as coined by Robert Lanza, MD.: "the attempt to explain the nature of the universe, its origins, its parameters, and what is really going on, requires an understanding of how the observer – our presence – plays a role. At first this may seem impossibly difficult, since much of awareness or consciousness and certainly its origins are still mysterious. But as we shall see, we can use what we know, and what we are increasingly discovering, to formulate models of the cosmos that make sense of things for the first time." (Biocentrism: How Life and Consciousness Are the Keys to Understanding the True Nature of the Universe. By Dr. Robert Lanza and Bob Berman: Ben Bella Books, 2009).

Which came first, the chicken or the egg? Essentially, Biocentrism claims that the universe comes from consciousness, not the other way around. If consciousness is, in fact, the source of our reality, it is reasonable that the belief-structure of personality (paradigm) is what determines whether there is *evolution* (definition: A gradual process in which something changes into a different and usually more complex or better form) or *devolution* (definition: 1. A descent through successive stages of time or a process. 2. Biological Degeneration.)

In the past, it has been the culture of death that determined our human condition, at times motivating our youth to take their lives through suicide and risk-taking, most recently demonstrated as mass school shootings. Revealing the nature of the *Battle of the Sexes* will also reveal the source of this repetitive electromagnetic conundrum called *heartlessness*. In the face of pandemic heartlessness, it is next to impossible for a loving soul to maintain a healthy Will to live; even so, pandemic depression is not our birthright! Fortunately, there is new information today that exposes many misunderstandings and serve to potentially motivate a willing soul to explore previously unimagined solutions.

Healing our own heartlessness (lack of electromagnetic reciprocity) is as simple as making a decision to go on living and feeling our own unique truth. For many of us, after having hushed the negative voice of disturbance that the *Battle of the Sexes* relentlessly produces, we may have difficulty feeling what we have been denying in the name of survival all this time. There is no formula that will apply to all people because Personal Sovereignty is unique and developing a reciprocal electromagnetic exchange will lead a soul toward custom-made solutions. Once you understand the tools that you were given at birth, you will quite naturally want to activate your magnetism to draw experiences that thrill your heart and make the cells of your body hum with life-force, this is a very good formula for supporting our ongoing Will to live.

The Will to live is a force of nature.

OVERVIEW OF CHAPTER ONE:

1. Earth (Gaia) is our primary element that is powered by the sun (Helios).

2. The human Light Body is a microcosm of the same electromagnetic relationship shared between the sun and earth.

3. Bio-centrism is a quantum physics postulate that claims the universe was created by consciousness instead of consciousness arising from random biological events.

4. Today, it has been scientifically shown that the earth herself is responsive to humanity's collective, heartfelt emotions.

5. The Microzymian Principle has scientifically demonstrated how cosmic dust particles (the building blocks of all plant, blood and tissue on earth) are responsive to consciousness and not subject to death.

6. Pleomorphism is the ability of a human cell to mutate into a morbid agent of death or mutate adaptations that further support life.

CHAPTER 2

HELIOS

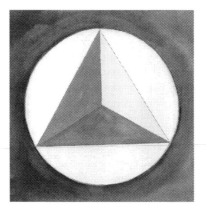

ELEMENT FIRE

The closest symbol mankind has to actually representing an Almighty God on this sphere of death and war is our local star, named Helios by ancient Greeks. Helios is the master of our Solar System simply because this star is the most essential presence in our daily lives, beside the earth herself! Rulers and kingdoms come and go, but reverence for this only leads to slavery or a lack of sovereignty (personal freedom). The *Principle of Pangasm* is not a religion, nor does this information lend itself to the occult, instead, this principle is detailing the pathway to personal sovereignty that is founded upon the precepts of Free Will. What an individual believes to be true constitutes a unique and evolving perfection that is their 'Personality' and Personal Sovereignty (the right for an adult to make his/her own decisions, as long as he/she does not harm self or the other) is our birthright.

This revolutionary paradigm does not put one in a position of having to oppose religion or the occult. In fact, this principle is all-inclusive with the exception of those who use violence as a solution. As to what this does or does not mean to you, will be determined by you and you alone.

What gives a thinking person the power to FEEL the truth? It is the nature of the human magnetic field to be the feeling part of us. We relate to this part of ourselves as Emotions and/or the human WILL. The truth is a living and dynamic presence of BEING that will set us free when we consecrate our heart to expressing our truth at all times. Unfortunately, in the past, speaking truth to power about the ongoing Battle of the Sexes has marginalized an entire class of human beings whose job it is to sound the sirens that are meant to warn us about chronic imbalance as a means of motivating the group to address this long-standing problem. Instead, the power structure of mankind has demonized, or criminalized this class of people to the point that this group, generally speaking, populate our prisons, asylums and fill the ranks of the homeless. Addiction is also a symptom of this unfortunate pattern that persistently creates the illusion of human garbage.

Today, in the United States, a common condition called "Bi-Polar Disorder" is suffered widely, even in our youth. Remember the example of how magnets repel one another when similarly polarized? Extreme emotions ping-ponging between highs and lows is the classic symptom of the ongoing Battle of the Sexes, and quite often, this pattern robs us of our integrity as the dysfunction of chronic imbalance captures our whole self. Mental disease or emotional disturbance is not our birthright, nor is it a manifestation of being bad; there is simply balance and imbalance; understanding the principle of electromagnetic bonding and pH is a super way to begin the life-affirming process of pangasm.

When chronic imbalance is deemed as *normal* the way to establish balance is rarely sought out. Even so, we are not bad people becoming good -- we simply suffer from a collective misunderstanding about the birthright that is innate to human personality. We have been provided for in the way of warmth, oxygen, plants, and water without fail…this is "Providence"; to the extent that we refuse providence is the measure to which we suffer. Providence is a broad term that means many things to many people, but the bottom line here is… Providence is the breath that feeds us every time we inhale; is the global breast that satisfies us every time we drink water; it is the seed that knows exactly what we need to eat, and, PROVIDENCE IS PATIENT. But, there is a limit to He/She's patience toward any personality willfully contributing to imbalance, injustice and self-destruction.

When one has been indoctrinated by the Battle of the Sexes, confusion replaces our ability to feel the truth and create peaceful situations that inspire our Will to live. In the current human condition, we are not to blame for our confusion even though it has been a long slow journey to this point in our journey of using devolution as a means of evolution. If a personality could gain "seemingly" magical powers enabling them to draw their heart's desire, there would be heartfelt gratitude, instead of denied desperation, neglect, abuse or self-destructiveness. I am not suggesting that being wealthy and having the ability to buy whatever your heart desires is all there is to happiness because without health, money holds little value. Being healthy and having our basic needs met is not a frivolous desire, nor is longing to be met by a desirable other, in a loving sexual relationship, a frivolous desire.

Helios represents the element of fire and is the Direct Current (DC) for the heavenly bodies that encircle this small star on the outskirts of the Milky Way galaxy. The sun's macrocosmic magnetic arms hold the 9 planets of our solar system in a paternal embrace keeping them safe from wandering off into the ethers of space. Recently, all the other planets have been going through magnetic pole shifts and there is much consensus that the earth is currently undergoing just such a transformation. The last time this happened on earth was 780,000 years ago, making this episode completely unmatched by any other event in modern history and beyond.[2] This interesting and stunning information is gathered by studying the magnetic fragments of lava. When lava solidifies, the magnetic particles point North helping scientists to record the timing of this regular global adjustment, which is shared equally by the other planets of the solar system.

Paleo-climatologists (those who study earth's past climates through various types of core sample studies) have recorded the Apocalyptic Earth Changes of the distant past (hundreds of millions of years) and have shown that mankind suffers major setbacks as a result of regular earth changes, presenting us with countless forms of death that will be referred to here as *INTIMIDATING FORM*. Helios and Gaia can be entirely intimidating to mankind, especially when Gaia lets down her magnetic field and allows Helios to shoot solar flares directly to the earth's surface. This is a serious level of intimidating form that has spurred heated international debate about whether or not mankind is the cause of "Global Warming". Generally, the earth's magnetic field shields us from the sun's radiation, however, today, earth's magnetic field is heading for, or at, magnetic minimum which is one of the reasons the earth is heating up to the point of having a global Melt-Water event that has been escalating since the 1970's.

Helios has solar cycles that are approximately 22 years in duration while Gaia has a magnetic cycle that is estimated to be a 4 thousand year cycle. The last time earth was at "Magnetic Maximum" (the opposite of today's Magnetic Minimum) was 2 thousand years ago – marking the beginning of the Gregorian calendar that Western societies use to keep time. (*The Earth's Magnetic Field: it's history, origin, and planetary perspective*" by, Ronald T. Merrill, M.W. McElhinny)

---

2   A geomagnetic reversal is a change in the orientation of Earth's magnetic field such that the positions of magnetic north and magnetic south become interchanged. These events often involve an extended decline in field strength followed by a rapid recovery after the new orientation has been established. These events occur on a scale of tens of thousands of years or longer, with the latest one occurring 780,000 years ago.

Helios is about to enter into another Solar Maximum event that is scheduled to peak in 2012/2013. The previous Solar Maximum event blew all of the past solar emission records off of the table! This last cycle, (cycle number 23) was supposed to end around 2001, but continued to emit significant, record-breaking amounts of solar wind (electromagnetic particles) well into 2003. Solar storms create solar winds that heat the earth's core for 5 to 7 years past the peak event itself, helping earth's battery to be re-charged to maintain her electromagnetic dynamo and essentially helps Gaia to maintain a viable magnetic field. When the sun increases it's output, (as it did during cycle 23), while the earth is also dropping the strength of her Magnetic Field to Magnetic Minimum, solar-radiation heats the interior causing the polar ice-caps and glaciers to melt, as well as, delivering doses of radiation to all life-forms mutating entirely new plant and animal species.

An interesting result of historical studies that compile solar output in connection to war and political unrest, proves that solar storms coincide with the outbreak of war, earthquakes, volcanic activation, changing jet streams, extreme weather and pandemic levels of depression and/or aggression, hence increased warfare (*Solar Rain*", by Mitch Battros.) Intimidating Form comes in all shapes and sizes on earth and on any given day, tens of thousands of people are dying. Some dare to dream of a day when these horrors cease to exist. In ancient Mesopotamia, where the original books of the Bible were first written, many prophecies were set into the Western human psyche about death and immortality that have guided the course of Western civilization. In First Corinthians 5:1, the Apostle Paul wrote: "Behold, I shew you a mystery; we shall not all sleep, but shall all be changed. In a moment, in the twinkling of an eye, at the last trump: for the trumpet shall sound, and the dead shall be raised incorruptible, and we shall be changed. For this corruptible must put on incorruption, and this mortal must put on immortality. So when this corruptible shall have put on incorruption, and this mortal shall have put on immortality, then shall be brought to pass the saying that is written: Death is swallowed up in victory. O death, where is thy sting? O grave, where is thy victory? The sting of death is sin; and the strength of sin is the law."

In the book of Revelation, the Apostle John wrote about the glorious future of man as described by a divine being that spoke to him: "Behold, the tabernacle of God is with men, and he will dwell with them, and they shall be his people, and God himself shall be with them, and be their God. And God shall wipe away all tears from their eyes; and there shall be no more death, neither sorrow, nor crying, neither shall there be any more pain: for the former things are passed away" (*The Bible - The book of Revelation*: 21:3)

Equally, in the Book of Revelations, there is much written about the "*End-times*" of mankind that many refer to as "*Christian Fire and Brimstone*". These statements prophesize about what will happen to the "un-redeemed or un-repentant sinner". As we can see today, many Christians, Jews and Muslims are at war, and they all believe the world is experiencing the end-times referred to as "*Armageddon*" or the "*Rapture*". Now, in 2010, there is much discussion about the year 2012 as being the next date that is predicted to be the day of destruction for modern society. My point here is that self-fulfilling prophecy places a great influence upon the hearts and minds of men and women, to the point of causing long-standing religious ideas to take on physical form. Many unfortunate events have occurred behind fervent religious ideas that have led to the persecution and genocide of whole populations. Today is no exception, even in modern times with our scientific insight there is great movement toward the finding of a scapegoat for all the evil that is amongst us!

According to the Maya, the end-date of their calendar (12/21/2012) predicts "*THE END OF THE WORLD AS WE KNOW IT.*" The keen astronomical records of the Maya align with those of the ancient Egyptians, as archeology reveals that pyramids exist in all regions on earth and speak to modern man of long-standing astronomical cycles and correlating earth changes. In Adrian Gilbert's book "*Signs in the Sky*", he clearly makes a case that one of the functions of the largest pyramid in the Egyptian Giza complex points to the 26,000-year precession-cycle of the constellation Orion. This alignment with the Constellation Orion is an astronomical timepiece that shows the year 2000 as the beginning of a New Age upon the earth; this also aligns with the Star-Gate event presented by the Mayan astronomical records as peaking during the Solstice of 2012.

As we can clearly see, today the earth is experiencing a Melt Water event that is changing the normal weather patterns as well as motivating nations around the world to begin the conversation about the advent of Global Warming and whether or not mankind is responsible for this intimidating transformation. As a result of this global conversation, the human race has, and is experiencing a New Age of international interaction that will one day align the nations of the world to end the advent of wars between nations as a result of heightened awareness and cooperation. This has been a long-standing prayer held in the hearts of millions, if not billions of souls down through the ages.

When we speak of saving our planet, to a large extent we mean saving the Biosphere that supports our lifeline: oxygen, water and plants. Understanding that the sun is the major driver of the earth's climatic condition puts extra emphasis upon the usually predictable star that is the center of our Solar System. As previously mentioned, solar activity can create a microburst and wipe out an entire city block within minutes…this is entirely intimidating; Helios, as a mad daddy patriarch in the sky, actually aligns with many of the ancient and modern religious attitudes about a patriarchal God. Equally, earth's unpredictable and harsh moods are facets of life that all humans have attempted to control forever, while many people personify nature as a mother that punishes. Today, thanks to the GOES satellite observations, we know that the earth is like a mother that is responsive to her creation in loving and protective ways. It is also reasonable to assume that the sun is equally aware of the earthly events and the ways of humanity.

As I learn more about my own body, I have come to find out that humans have an energetic body that can change their physical condition in an instant ("form follows energy" – quote from Einstein). Science has shown how positive thinking can actually help the body heal much faster, but why has positive thinking failed to stop war, neglect, abuse or disease? As the sun and earth have an energetic relationship that I like to relate to as romantic, so do human beings have an energetic Light Body that has a male (yang) part and a female (yin) part. The brain is the electric part (yang/masculine) and our body is the magnetic part (yin/feminine). Today, the human Light Body is a proven scientific fact, whereas, in the past this was considered a metaphysical theory that was treated with great skepticism. Our Light Body is so wonderful I would need to write a much longer book to describe its wonders!

All vibrating things in this world have their own "natural" frequency, and human brain waves undergo fluctuations just as the earth's Schumann Frequency is the measurement of her currently rising frequency…something like a fever. When a thing is subjected to an external force that makes it vibrate at a frequency it vibes with the most, the thing responds by vibrating at the maximum amplitude (energy). This phenomenon manifests throughout the universe. This natural frequency of that thing or body is known as its "resonating" or "resonant" frequency, and the phenomenon is known as "Resonance".

The basic function of our Light Body is to maintain a resonant frequency of electromagnetic exchange referred to here as electromagnetic "*RECIPROCITY*". This keeps the dense physical body vital and healthy, only if the electric part is reciprocal (freely exchanging properties) with the magnetic part in our heart. However, the Human Condition disengages our electromagnetic reciprocity at an early age, as discussed in the 4th chapter that discusses the element Ether. A vibrant electro-magnetic exchange should be occuring in our heart, which is the organ that connects heaven and earth in the center of our being. This being the case, then we can heal any injury, prevent disease, become immune to toxins and possess many other seemingly super-human qualities as demonstrated by Indigo Children.

The influx of a new genetic class of human beings, that have been identified as *"Indigo Children"*, possess super-human traits such as immunity to disease and heightened Extra-sensory Perceptions (ESP.) This advanced population of people are coming in upon the larger populations of average people helping to uplift the vibratory frequency of the masses.[3]

During episodes of heightened species evolution, the newly emergent hybrid of the dominant species comes in and begins to develop a critical mass of presence capable of evolving the entire species to the higher level of adaptation; in essence, the resonant frequency of this population stimulates the elder generations to also rise in frequency. This addition to our species, in combination with our increasing technological ability, makes for a vital shift in human consciousness, especially in regard to health and longevity.

If one is in balance mentally and emotionally, then the Will to Live is ever-present, making it much more likely that one will also be a vital

---

3   During the later part of the Seventies a woman called Nancy Ann Tappe noticed a change taking place in the colour of Children's auras. She did a lot of work in China and taught at the University of San Diego. As part of her research and study she published a book in 1982 called Understanding Your Life Through Color. In that, this is where the first mention of indigo is talked about. Lee Carol and Jan Tober, authors of The Indigo Children and Indigo Celebration presented Tappe's research on varying colours of the aura. Tappe recognized that after 1980 about 80% of the babies being born had this aura around them that she equated to their life mission and their life colour. It was what she called Indigo. As of 1990 she realized that there were about 90% being born. Indigo is the colour of the third eye chakra, which is an energy centre inside the head located between the two eyebrows. This chakra regulates clairvoyance, or the ability to see energy, visions and spirits, so many of the Indigo Children are classed as clairvoyant. Nancy was able to carry out this unique research because she has a medical diagnosis of Synesthesia. That's where two neurological systems become crossed so that the senses get reversed. She actually sees like a Kirlian camera. What seems to be her dysfunction has ended up being a great gift.

and contributing part of the collective reality we ALL share. Today, we are transforming rapidly together through the communication revolution that is transmitting the knowledge about revolutionary scientific breakthroughs like the *Microzymian Principle*. The dust that comprises our body is as essential as our Light Body when it comes to maintaining health. The human Light Body is an amazing vehicle once it becomes activated. The ancient Hebrew called the Light Body the *"Chariot"* or *"Merkabah"*, The Urantia Book calls it the *"Chariot of the Blue Flame"* because it is the all-encompassing energetic vessel from which the human form springs.

Ancient Chinese Tantrica priestesses were able to live hundreds of years longer than their fellow countrymen because they understood the life-giving properties of a reciprocal Light Body and understood how to activate it through their sexuality. However, once the electromagnetic matrix is interrupted and the electric is not reciprocating with the magnetic, then the yin and the yang fall apart. Heart attacks and mental disease are the tip of the iceberg when it comes to humanity's demonstration of the current Human Condition as fostered by the Battle of the Sexes.

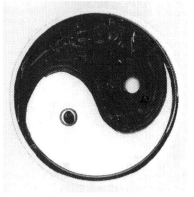

YINYANG'

Look again at the yinyang diagram above, and see that there are more than just male and female at play in this because there are four parts to the yin/yang matrix. This 4-part matrix (the two fish, plus the black circle and white circle) is the same design as the human heart and represents the 4 parts of Personality, North, South, East and West or CROWN (consciousness), ROOT (emotions), HEART (personality) and BODY (responsive cosmic dust and water). As self-aware animals, we maintain a cellular form that reflects the energetic matrix of the yin/yang. In order to hum with the frequency of life, it is important to be firing on all 4 cylinders, so to speak. The healing process advocated by the *Principle of Pangasm* leads the willing into a gathering of self, a re-capitulation of our electromagnetic ether in a way that makes a personality energetically sustainable. In this way, our intimate relationship with our own physical form becomes a dynamic relationship capable of delivering orgasmic rapture at Will.

Recent scientific studies will help us relate to our Light Body so we can make sense of the goals and techniques of Pangasm. The superhuman influence that an aligned personality has upon its own incarnate body liberates that person to relate to his/her body as a magical vessel with a language all of its own, complete with unique solutions for each and every body. There is no other heart in the Universe that is like your own, which is why the principle before you does not attempt to define your goals for you. The mysterious magnetic aspect of our being, the human Will, has in the past, been relegated to shamans and priests, but now it is within the realm of science and exposing the truth about the Laws of Nature will give many tools to those who wish to establish perfect health and longevity, not to mention, oodles of intimacy with the 'other'.

Why is mankind not utilizing its birthright of perfect health within a responsive and supportive environment?

We have a misunderstanding about the magnetic aspect of our human Will.

Today, science is suggesting that the Homo-Sapien has slowed in evolutionary progress. Does this mean the end of the Homo-Sapien? Recent studies have shown that chimpanzees are evolving at a faster rate than we are. Does this mean that the movie the "Planet of the

Apes" is prophetic? I suppose if we insist on refusing the hand of Providence, we deserve to be the familiars of the apes!

Oh, yes, all we have ever known about the hand of providence was the slapping part, instead of the nurturing part. Did I leave that part out? Under the influence of *The Battle of the Sexes*, intimidating form is our constant companion, therefore: stress is the *Human Condition*. How do we create Intimidating Form? How do we continually attract unwanted experiences? Understanding the role of human magnetism is key to creating what one desires. Understanding our biology and also learning about the 5 elements that comprise all physical form on earth is essential to creating true Free Will. Without health, life becomes a drudgery of existence. Intimidating form can simply be an unresponsive body, such as disease, the ugliness of aging, impotency, frigidity or intimidating form can be violence from others, threat of jail, homelessness, addiction, debility/dependency....etc.

It is from our personality that our decision-making stems. This is the place no other personality has access to other than you. From our inner world we create our unique reality. To the extent that we are creating realities we did not think we created, but instead were put upon us from the outer world is the extent to which we will persistently be under the illusion that we are under the control of others. However, as I studied the difference between the inner world and the outer world, I could see that the outer world was responding to what I believe in ways that frightened me! Truly, when I learned about how very powerful I actually am I sat on my hands for a time, terrified by how much denial had influenced my decisions and fully well-knowing that I did not consciously want to continue creating crisis, estrangement or poor health! From this place, I began to understand the true nature of Personal Sovereignty and have a healthy respect for the power that denial has to form my Personality and, therefore, all of my experiences.

If you really contemplate the ramifications of the Laws of Nature, you will begin to see how far reaching are the implications of a universe that is responsive to personality. You will come to realize that the part of divinity that you hold in your human heart is a miracle, even magical. I dare say that the *Principle of Pangasm* is a handbook for becoming a magical persona that is capable of changing the world by simply telling one's truth and harboring aligned desire. The important role that truth-telling has in helping us create balanced and sustainable experiences, rather than scenarios that further serve to re-enforce self-doubt, self-rejection and systemic guilt, is all-encompassing. In order to keep from making anyone feel guilt when they contemplate this, I have chosen to expose this problem, that we all inherited, through describing the electromagnetic patterns that continually convince our personality to subvert the truth out of a very reasonable survival terror. Once we all understand that we were all indoctrinated into a false-hood, we could begin to then take responsibility to the extent of making moral choices from a place of understanding true Free Will.

The human heart is more than just a physiological organ. Heart's role in holding our parts together is seemingly super-human. I will devote an entire chapter (chapter 5) to describing the qualities of the human heart as a way of giving insight to the relationship between the spiritual realm of the **4th dimension** (our unique inner world) and the physical realm of the **5th dimension** (the Five Elements of density). Through simple awareness we have a greater influence upon all aspects of our life that were not offered by the dominant paradigm of the Battle of the Sexes. (*Note: this reference to various dimensions is used to help differentiate the parts of personality and the elemental reality that responds to personality and may not necessarily align with other uses of these terms*).

As a result of aligning the 4 parts of personality (Father/electric, Mother/magnetic, Daughter/heart and Son/body) with the 5 elements of nature, (earth, fire, water, ether and air) one can achieve super-human levels of Personal Sovereignty powered by the quantum energetic force of orgasm. A Light Body is no longer a metaphysical concept to be revealed only by metaphysical teachers. It is now possible to photograph the electromagnetic part of us and reveal whether or not there is a full spectrum of color capable of maintaining a full spectrum of vibration. The game of Pangasm (chapter 7) is not only a fun way to align these mysterious parts of our personality, but it is also a great learning experience that will make us aware of what these parts feel like and how they operate in the 'other'.

As many of us already know, emotional disturbance and mental disease are becoming quite common-place, while drugging these parts as a way of creating balance between these parts of self, only postpones the disturbance! Eventually these parts need to come out from under this kind of pressure and misunderstanding to be integrated. This process is made more practical when the suffering individual comes into awareness about what these parts are and what their nature is. This is a way of empowering the disturbed person to feel as though he or she has the ability to recover without becoming dependent upon drugs or even other people. No outside person has the ability to understand our inner world better than we do. According to the *Principle of Pangasm*, we have more options for creating balance through integrating our inner world to form an aligned prayer about what it is we desire from life. In this way, we become empowered to create a life worth living that is full of meaning and value. Meanwhile, we are living in a highly charged and volatile reality that is filled with intimidating form and we need clarity about our whole self…the conscious parts as well as the denied parts. We cannot access personal power by creating further blame or shame about being caught within the dominant paradigm of the Battle of the Sexes.

As the GOES satellites revealed, the earth is responsive to our collective emotions, and it goes to reason that the sun is also intimately involved with all life in this solar system. Imagine the earth responding to the collective grief triggered by the toppling of the World Trade Center on September 11, 2001! Understanding that the earth is highly aware and responsive opens our minds and hearts to begin considering that the sun is also intimately aware of the creation that it directly affects as the *Direct Current* (DC) for this solar system. As it is, the sun is the primary driver of the earth's atmospheric composition. It is the moods of Helios that maintains our lifeline and it is reasonable to suspect that the electromagnetic relationship between the sun and the earth aligns with and supports the responsiveness characterized by the elements. "As it is within, so it is without". The microcosmic realm replicates the macrocosmic realm and if a cell in our body is capable of mutating into a morbid form (such as cancer, yeast, mold or fungi) and killing our entire body, it is also possible that the human personality can be considered a cell in the macrocosmic body of the universe. In essence, our influence upon our own personal life and the outer world is far greater than we ever previously imagined as a race of sentient beings with Free Will.

As I try to describe the presence of the sun to be a cognizant being that has the ability to wipe out mankind with one earth directed solar flare, or even to decide to not emit any energy what-so-ever. I can only imagine that you wonder if I have lost my ever-lov'in mind! All I can say is that the wonders of Helios have only been the stuff of ancient fairy-tales or earth-based religions that originated all religions, and, tell you unabashedly that Helios will reveal many things to us in the upcoming months and years, which is only possible because we now live in this new age of heightened awareness and communication. As prophesied by ancient religious text, the cosmos will work in alignment with an almighty God to help mankind rise to the heights of love or the depths of despair depending upon the collective paradigm. Many religions were created as a way of convincing humanity to choose love and honesty over corruption. We can hardly blame religion as the cause of mankind's corrupt state, even though religion has been used to unfairly control large groups of people for nefarious reasons in the past.

Today, self-fulfilling prophecies of apocalyptic destruction fill the masses with horrible predictions about God's Will for them based upon the embrace of concepts such as original sin (mankind's basic belief that men and women are intrinsically evil). It only makes sense that the earth and sun have responded to the cries of the multitudes to end our world through major earth-change upheavals in the past.

OVERVIEW OF CHAPTER TWO:

1. Our energetic model is the YinYang symbol and is also a physiological representation of the human heart.

2. The human heart is what holds the metaphysical and the physical together as human personality. It is the organ that synthesizes our inner realm and outer realm, aligning heaven and earth as a unified Personality capable of creating bio-spiritual balance.

3. Through scientific evidence, it has been shown that the earth is responsive to human sentiment. It is postulated by the Principle of Pangasm that, *the sun is as responsive as the earth*, since the symbiotic energetic relationship that they share, as the Alternating Current (AC) of the root and the Direct Current (DC) of the crown, is as inseparable as that of the energetic dynamo symbolized by the yinyang.

4. The Star-Gate event is a regular astronomical occurrence that follows the earth's 26,000 year *Precession Cycle*.

5. It is in alignment with the *LAWS OF NATURE* that mankind can play a role in determining what the new climate will be through evolving a new dominant paradigm aligned with life, instead of death.

CHAPTER 3

ELEMENT WATER

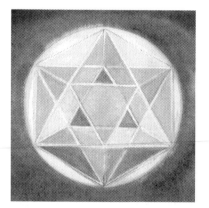

H2O – HOH

Got Water? Water (HOH or H2O) is the magic ingredient for life on earth. We are about 80% water in this holographic maze of microtubules that make up our highly mutable, evolutionary body. Our bodies demonstrate our current paradigm by representing our entire reality (past and present) as manifest in the flesh. But, we treat our flesh as if it were some embarrassing demon that needs to be concealed, as well as, being ashamed of our bodily functions, etc. The disposable body syndrome is the long-standing manifestation of the Battle of the Sexes and plays havoc with our Will to live. When the body's systems malfunction, it can be traumatic and rapid, while, for some, the body refuses to die after a long and debilitated state and languishes in extreme forms of debility for decades. A terribly slow death shows how a body, if not interrupted by disease, accidents or suicide/murder, can slowly decline in vibratory frequency and fall apart on a gradual cellular level. This is another example of constant

Intimidating Form and is a constant presence that must be denied in favor of living.

This denied survival terror flip flops between terror and rage constantly present during the ups and downs, the ins and outs of daily life. For the most part this form of stress is a rational way to deal with intimidating form, because mankind has not known that the Laws of Nature are in absolute service of what a personality believes to be true about reality. Our collective paradigm has created a reality based upon intimidating form that is sincerely considered to be beyond our control. Truly we did not understand the extent to which we had true Free Will. In the case of the element water, it perhaps demonstrates the most impressive form of responsiveness to consciousness.

My hero, Dr. Masaru Emoto, published a book called "*The Message From Water*" (Hado Publishing) detailing the conscious nature of water using photographic evidence. In his study, Dr. Emoto conducted microphotography of frozen water crystals before and after the water was exposed to different forms of stimulus. This was done by freezing a water sample and photographing its frozen, crystalline geometry, and then, thawing the water and exposing it to music, art, written words and even prayer. Once the water was influenced by one of these stimuli, it would be re-frozen and photographed again. What Dr. Emoto discovered is the magical and responsive nature of water, both within and without.

"When water freezes it becomes crystallized, and at the moment right before it returns to its liquid form (with a rise in temperature between 5C and 0C) it creates a gaseous matrix that is identical to the Chinese symbol for water." (See the following photograph) The Chinese symbol for water is universally part of the geometrical expression of all water as it is undergoing temperature transition from ice to liquid.

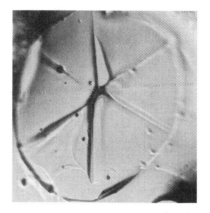

'Water that is forming the Chinese symbol for water'

The following two photographs are of a water sample taken from a river in Japan, before and after Reverend Kato of the Jyuhouin Temple of Omiya City offered prayers at the water's edge.

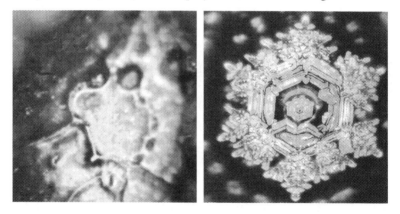

This next experiment was repeated with a sample of Tokyo tap water, except this time Dr. Emoto made requests of 500 different people from different locations to send prayers to and for this water sample. Dr. Emoto requested from the participants of this experiment that the prayers specifically send "Chi and soul of love….and, to wish that the water should become clean," The results of this are quite stunningly beautiful!

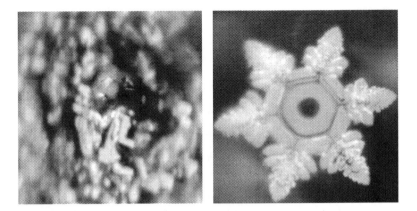

For more information about Dr. Emoto's books and studies go to www. hadousa.net. or www.hadoeurope.net

The consciousness that water possesses demonstrates the magic that the world around us is vibrating. In essence, what we are witnessing in these pictures is the absolute responsiveness of the unified 9th dimensional reality, where the 5 elements (in this case, water) are demonstrating alignment with the 4 parts of personality (Spirit, Will, Heart and Body). All water has consciousness that is responsive and is the same type of responsiveness that originates from the Feminine Principle of magnetism.

Dr. Emoto has published extensive photographic evidence of the consciousness that water possesses in a series of books, starting with *'The Message From Water'*. I personally feel as though Dr. Emoto has made it possible to demonstrate that we do have Free Will, by suggesting that the Universal Law of Personality is perfectly supported by that which we are made of and that which surrounds us.

When I first witnessed this evidence, I was equally amazed and ashamed. I was ashamed to realize that prayer is effective, as witnessed by the instant transformation of water, but somehow not for me. Faced with the evidence that I can purify all the water in my body by simply saying or thinking the words: "I now purify all the water in my body", I had to ask myself why was I experiencing heartbreaking difficulties in any area of my life…health, family, finance or romance? Literally, I felt like a spiritual cripple when I grasped this scientific truth. Why was I struggling if this is true of Creation? Lord knows I have prayed feverishly for some relief while spending many inspired moments worshipping my understanding of God. As to whether or not I was able to receive the blessings I asked for was dependent upon my ability to accept PROVIDENCE as the basis of the physical world.

As we witness the consciousness that drops of water exhibit, it is natural to assume that all life containing electromagnetic frequency has some form of consciousness that responds to its environment. Personality is spiritual because humans harbor a self-awareness that is capable of moral decision-making. This type of spiritual prerogative has its own electromagnetic method of influencing self and the outer world that is keyed to what that person believes about self and the other/outer world.

The plant populations on Earth possess tremendous telepathic properties that demonstrate responsiveness to personality, much as the water does in Dr. Emoto's study. In a famous study called "*The Secret Life of Plants*", (by Peter Tompkins and Christopher Bird) it was conclusively proven that plants of all kinds respond to human consciousness. Interestingly enough, plants can and will respond to a person that is in a distant location from the plant. For instance, in my own life, as a farmer and forester, I have had success keeping jungle trails open by meditating on the plants that border this trail and ask them not to grow across this. As long as I regularly asked this of the plants, they responded positively by keeping the trail open. Also, in recent years, I have had success with planting trees and groundcover through prayer. That's right, you can pray a tree into existence! Someday, I will be teaching more about the developing spiritual methods of reforestation and farming that will make a difference in our ongoing environmental crisis that is currently poised to make deserts where there were once forests, rivers and lakes.

As we witness these properties in the microcosmic realm of molecules, plants, animals and people, it is natural to draw the conclusion that the macrocosmic realm of planets and stars also possess consciousness that is responsive to personality. Indeed, it seems only natural that all the heavenly bodies that constitute a Universe are personified as sentient Beings with prerogative (Free Will) of their own. I believe Gaia has Free Will and is making drastic earth changes at this time to create balance from the gross imbalance that has emerged down through the ages as a result of humanity's dominant paradigm. As we begin to uncover the mystery of Mars, and how this nearby planet lost its ambient atmosphere when there obviously was one in the past, it is more than likely that we will discover that we destroyed that delicate atmosphere, prior to evolving on the earth. As we are poised to destroy our own atmospheric composition on the earth, through nuclear war, carbon emissions and deforestation, it is possible to jog our collective memory and make life-confirming decisions this time. Truly, our world media is doing a good job of exposing the truth of the human condition in ways that could lead to amazing developments that inspire human beings to allow one another to live in peace and Free Will.

Solar flare activity on the sun can change the ambient atmosphere of the earth because Helios has the ability to help Gaia maintain, and, even enhance our ambient atmosphere or alter it in ways that may be deadly to entire species such as dinosaurs. Even with comets and asteroids present in and around our solar system (such as the asteroid Apophos approaching earth in 2039), the sun is able to alter their orientation in a way that could send them to earth or deflect them. Our sun is an ever-present authority figure that could support our collective Will to live or support our collective Will to end it already!

There is much evidence to suggest that highly evolved civilizations have existed on Gaia in the past and scientific consensus states that earth changes destroyed these ancient civilizations, as well as some modern ones (past 10,000 years). Through the study of Paleo-climatology, core sample comparisons have begun to establish the record of past climate models, helping us realize that the earth and sun have collaborated to establish Ice Age cycles in the past. These were brought about by the cycles of earth's magnetic field variable, her axis and tilt, whether or not Gaia is in an elliptical orbit to the sun or a circular one, as well as extra-terrestrial events such as gamma ray blasts, asteroids, comets and especially the moods of Helios (CME's --- Coronal Mass Ejections).

The sun's intensity is the most influential extra-terrestrial climate driver of our atmospheric composition because Helios is our astronomical god in that he determines our existence by his nature and his moods. Helios is a BEING among other stars as the stars verify in their perfect display of individuality and collective alignment. I have a deep appreciation for the climatic stasis provided by Helios and Gaia on a daily basis. Most of the time I feel blessed to be in a body on earth and know this would not be true if it were not for the symbiotic relationship of agreement between the sun and earth that has given our world the stability necessary to provide for our every need as we evolve.

The current *MELT-WATER* event that is happening on earth is the precursor to a new climate. As fellow earthlings it will be helpful for us to have a sense of what pattern earth-changes have previously followed while at the same time considering the aspect of Free Will in regard to our future. Freedom is a relative issue depending upon where one may live, what religion is embraced, what family we belong to and how honest one may choose to be. The Christian term *"The truth shall set you free"* is highly revered by Westerners yet sufficiently marginalized by the symptoms of the Battle of the Sexes; nonetheless, all humans crave freedom. The fact that we live in groups makes our destiny a collective issue as well as an issue of individual choice. Regardless of the self-destructive patterns of humanity, it is possible to experience our own life-affirming reality by simply learning what tools we have to work with.

Learning about the solar system is as important as learning about our cellular biology when it comes to attaining and maintaining balance and asking for what we desire from a responsive Creation. I believe that humanity has much more influence upon the sun and earth than we ever dreamt possible because of the physical and metaphysical connections that make our creation much more personal and responsive than ever before contemplated. As mentioned previously, there is scientific evidence that the emotional energy of mankind does have a quantitative affect on the earth's magnetic field...our planetary shield. You and I have far greater degrees of influence over our own body and world at large, and therefore, capable of dreaming up a more favorable reality. We can simply do this by aligning our heart with life and agreeing on this with one another.

The empires that collapsed in the past did so because the populations had developed a collective agreement-field as a result of universal experiences based upon experiencing and observing the linear 3rd dimension. Collective agreements like "death is inevitable", "death is God's Will for us", "the nature of the animal kingdom is all there is to earth reality", "the spirit is willing, but the flesh is weak", etc, etc, etc...these thought-forms only serve to keep the 3rd dimension as a dead-end trap for one and all, existing for millennia unchallenged right up to the point when the group achieves a quantum presence and consciousness; this is where we currently find ourselves. When any group adopts the Battle of the Sexes as their dominant paradigm, as humanity universally does, their collective sexual essence builds on the foundation of death, inevitably causing the collapse of the social group according to their own self-fulfilling prophecies that perpetuate death. As a result of this group death-urge, the earth and sun move in unity to support this quantum collective concept by creating the reality the group was projecting. At regular intervals the earth and sun move in concert to erase all trace of our existence in accordance with our Free Will. As archeologists uncover the past, we continually find evidence of highly advanced civilizations that had left records of timelines pointing to these cyclical apocalyptic epochs, also known as Star-Gate.

As archeology uncovers ancient text and interprets the pyramids from around the world, there appears to be an aligned statement

Lori S. Dante

about the ramifications of the current Star-Gate as being an event that includes the entirety of the Milky Way galaxy. Thanks to major discovery in the field of Astronomy, we are now able to verify that we, as a planet and larger galaxy, are undergoing a significant shift in the heavens that is having a substantial affect upon the resonant frequency of the earth by making it rise significantly.

Both the ancient Maya and the Ancient Egyptians point to the 26,000-year precession cycle of the Constellation of Orion as an astronomical timekeeper registering this Star-Gate cycle that is currently ushering in a New Age on the earth ('*Signs in the Sky*' by, Adrien Gilbert). Through the study of ancient text and pyramids, much has come to light about the recurring patterns of collapsing civilizations which correlate with the astronomical Star-Gate events that are being predicted by the Western and Mayan calendars, as well as the Egyptian pyramids (among others).

All around the world people are deciphering the meaning of these symbolic messages. As we approach Star-Gate considering the implications of Free Will, (in regard to earth changes, such as, whether or not we have a choice about our climate). It's possible for us to achieve a collective agreement field that is melded into one voice about what we wish to set into motion for the next 26,000-year go-around Orion. We have, in all times past, held a universal belief about the inevitability of physical death, regardless of the seemingly immortal yogi's among us. By studying these regular patterns, it seems as though the dominant paradigm of the *Battle of the Sexes* contributes to the collapse of major societies as a reflection of what we continually do to our own individual physical body. Patterned un-sustainability is continually forcing the psyche of mankind to revert to hopeless ideas that support *Death Consciousness* (referred to here as D-Con) in such a way as it permeates our religious indoctrination and is considered fact.

We can plainly see that the water of earth is completely supportive of what it is we believe and it goes to reason that when mankind develops a whole-hearted agreement that reality is predatory, violent and deadly, then the elements provide these particular self-fulfilling prophecies of the group. After all is said and done, the celestial bodies that bore us are also responsive to personality, reaching from the level of the Universe (macrocosm) to the individual cell (microcosm). We are blessed with the ability to live or the ability to destroy what we have created, including our own selves, or, we could evolve our God concept to include absolute health that chooses not to over-ride the Will of another. Refusing violence and death as a solution, is a good start when addressing the Battle of the Sexes.

During the Star-Gate event the sun and earth ask the question "What is your desire dear children?" I can only imagine what it is like for them as they look and listen to the movements of men and women and see disparity, neglect, abuse, warfare and people having an orgy of lust around death and dying with all the inherent power trips mastered by the most brilliant among us!

"*What?*" says the earth and sun, "*You still believe that death is a solution to life? What a strange way to use the gift of Providence?!? Your wish is our command!*" Boom, shatter, crash, whoosh and collapse!!! Once again, the celestial Mother and Father of mankind move to mutate the species so that it can use the brain it was given in its next form.

Through simple decisions we can reconnect our Light Body to become reciprocal, in this way we may begin recovering our lost electromagnetic fullness. This is a dynamic life process that will give ever-greater integrity to our ability to create our heart's desire, instead of another crisis. In my own personal paradigm, it is possible to survive the self-destructive prayer of the group because I am not in denial of my life force. This prerogative I enjoy is available to one and all as long as the individual aligns their heart with life.

OVERVIEW OF CHAPTER THREE:

1. The element water is responsive to consciousness.

2. Plants are responsive to consciousness.

3. Indoctrination that denies the responsive aspect of the Laws of Nature can and does influence mankind's evolution in a way that causes chronic imbalance and un-sustainability (devolution) to be considered as "God's Will for us".

4. The human emotional body is the source of our Magnetic Ether or Chi. By denying our life force through erroneous thinking and false emotional illusions, we fall prey to the resultant Intimidating form that is designed to inform us of our denial, rather than to punish us for our misunderstandings.

5. Our bodies are a maze of microtubules (honeycomb tubules of mucous membranes and filled with water that conducts an electric current.) Pleomorphism gives our bodies the ability to shape-shift similar to the shape-shifting matrix of gaseous H_2O (water).

CHAPTER 4

ELEMENT ETHER

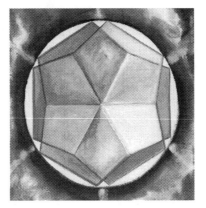

"GENII in a BOTTLE"

The element Ether (Chi) is the metaphysical substance of the human Light Body. We get our electric ether (silver Chi) from the sun and the magnetic ether (golden Chi) from the earth at all times. It is the function of the human heart to exchange the silver and gold Chi in and around our heart in order to maintain a viable Resonant Frequency. Unfortunately, for humanity, at this time, our ability to hold the ether present as a *reciprocal* Light Body has been crippled by the dominant paradigm...the Battle of the Sexes. The goal of *Pangasm* is to help us reconnect to our magnetic self in a way that completes our electromagnetic circuitry to become energetically sustainable.

It is the magnetic ether that holds the electric ether present in order to maintain a full spectrum of vibratory sound and color that a human Light Body is. Without a resonant frequency strong enough to maintain our cellular structure, our physical body begins to decay...we call this aging.

Just as we are influenced by the presence of other people, the earth is also influenced by the larger family of planets and stars, explaining why a Star-Gate is relative to the human family, as well as, relative to the family of stars that comprise our local Universe. According to this principle, our microcosmic human familial connections mirror the familial connections of the macrocosmic universal family of stars and planets. As it is within, so it is without. The pattern of the microcosm (microscopic cells, particles, electrons, neutrons, protons, etc.) mirrors that of the macrocosm (the cell that is the universe within a far-flung aggregate of other universes).

As stated previously, at this time earth's frequency is rising, as is her temperature; this phenomenon is in correlation with a magnetic pole shift that happens at regular intervals for the earth and all of the planets in our solar system. There are countless theories as to what will result from this transition we are all experiencing together as a *Melt-Water* event, however the *Principle of Pangasm* does not predict your future as much as it is suggesting that you align with your desired future as an individual and that we make an agreement about what we would like to create and experience as a collective group of spiritual beings, within the parameters of the Laws of Nature. With the advent of global communications, as in the world-wide-web, our species is having a global conversation about the future as we examine the past and consider the intimidating form that is triggering the collective survival terror. Negative emotions, such as survival terror, actually have a productive role to play in the transmutation of our race.

Having a Light Body is similar to having a "Genii in a bottle" when it comes to facilitating the Will of a human being. The human Will is our emotional self and it is also the part of us that selects our experiences and feels the result of our decision-making process; the mind, on the other hand, has the interpretive role ('*Right Use of Will*' by, *Ceanne De Rohan*). The Will chooses from all of the available choices that the mind is capable of perceiving, however, if the Will of man (the emotional body) is seen as a problem by its own mind, any number of experiences can occur depending upon the self-concept of the Personality. If the choices are limited to economic slavery, estrangement, aging, violence, war, disease and death, then the Will may lose the desire to live in such an anti-dynamic way of life. I find this rather perverse considering that we have been provided for freely, yet, we act as if everything is scarce and we are constantly in a rush to perform, only because we have a deadline…it's called mortality. We expect it and plan for it, prompting the Genii in our Bottle to fulfill our self-fulfilling prophecy…sometimes in slow, agonizing ways and very rapid at other times, depending upon the self-concept of the individual.

Since form follows energy, it only makes sense that refusing the hand of Providence would lead to countless moments of suffering and disillusionment. Knowing what we now know about water, dust, plants and our own biology, perhaps we could find more alternatives to the current trap that has most of the population enslaved to a few. How does our dominant paradigm force almost every person in the world to live under the threat of intimidating form as we try to be brave in the face of very frightening realities with ungrounded positive thinking? The Universal indoctrination process that affects every man, woman and child without fail, regardless of religion, ethnicity or location, is the dismantling of the electromagnetic part of our being as fostered by the Battle of the Sexes.

When all 4 parts of our personality (Spirit, Will, Heart and Body) are in alignment to go on living, then the 5 elements of Earth, Fire, Water, Ether and Air give us a capacity to create a reality that has not yet been realized on earth by modern men and women. Unfortunately, the indoctrination process that happens at birth for most of us begins with genital mutilation of boys in the Western societies, and genital mutilation of girls in the Eastern societies. Combine this with the disappearing use of human breast milk for infant nutrition and you have the anti-magical ingredients of violence and deprivation prior to the formation of the individual self-concept. These hallmarks of the

Human Condition do not directly affect all those that are born here, however, the number one indoctrination technique does happen to almost EVERY SINGLE human being, because the dominant paradigm of almost all people installs the 'death wish' as a result of a strange and unfortunate mass hypnosis.

The misunderstanding begins at a time in every child's life when their basic self-concept of their inner-world of personality (the 4th dimension) is developing in relation to their own body and outer world (the 5th dimension). At this time, the consciousness of the child reaches the stage where he or she can comprehend death and what this may mean for their own life and the lives of their loved ones. This is the moment that the dominant paradigm is installed for the lifetime of the child and the energetic consequence of this is terminal in scope, because the positive silver ether ceases to reciprocate with the negative golden ether. This holds the heart of this child within the confines of the dominant paradigm in a way that causes aging to begin at an early age...such as tooth decay and hyperactivity.

When a child first learns that they must die someday, no matter how "good" or "bad" they are, fear rises up from their root (the emotional self). Upon expressing this truthful response to the others about the specter of death, the child receives messages from all the adults and peers around them that say, "Everyone dies, so, stop being afraid because it won't do you any good! Acceptance is how to find peace with death and dying." This is the point where self-rejection (the rejection of the authentic emotions of survival terror becomes a subtle form of self-rejection) takes the position of authority. Regardless of the religious ideas that come in at this time to allay the natural fearful response of the child, the child must use his or her mind to inform the emotional self that its response to the threat of death should be different than fear. Very few children have the capacity to question authority at this juncture of development, making the imprint of death consciousness quite successful.

This subtle indoctrination is the wellspring of SELF-DOUBT and the source of the inevitable guilt that comes from thinking that our honest response to death is not quite right somehow!

Humanity's emotional spectrum is a vital source of our Life Force and it is from the depths of the earth that we freely receive the Golden Ether that is EMOTIONAL MAGNETIC ETHER. The nature of the mind and the emotions are different from one another, albeit, complementary in the action of living in the same way depicted by the yin/yang symbol. However, when the emotional self is disabled by the mind informing it that its emotional response is wrong, a subtle shift occurs that causes the mind to take over both positions of Spirit (positive-polarity) and Will (negative-polarity/emotions), thus creating a positive/positive or a negative/negative magnetic conundrum that constitutes the paradoxical Battle of the Sexes.

When positive does not sex with negative, the vibration collapses in on itself as demonstrated by the declining vibratory frequency of the aged, and the predictable and eventual corruption that leads societies to collapse. In a reciprocal Light Body there is free exchange of the dark magnetic Chi and the electric Chi so that the vibratory presence, known as resonance, allows the space for the personality to remain open, rather than creating a vacuum of self that collapses in upon itself.

As a result of the universal indoctrination process, the mind takes over the role of the emotional body in a relationship that mimics that of a master and slave, since the mind is attempting to control the emotional nature (this is especially acute when there is chronic imbalance). The emotions are the only means the individual has of feeling their own truth, so if we must rely upon our mind to discern the truth we will be eliminating the part of ourselves that can feel our truth, as well as lose the power to move magnetic ether to our heart from the depths of the earth. Many people become so disoriented by this that they go to others for information about what is true and what isn't true...we call this religion and/or psychiatry.

The emotional self is the selective part of personality and is the human WILL, our root. In a reciprocal state, the personality imagines the possibilities that life has to offer, inspiring the emotions to rise up and express the Will's desire for the imagined experience that the Will selects. When the magnetic essence of emotional response fills our heart, then East and West utter the 'Heart Song'...informing Creation of the Will's choice. As a result of this aligned prayer of desire, the Body becomes real. It is desire that chooses the individual reality, which is why it is called our HUMAN WILL. These parts of our self are a magical gift when they are reciprocal in the organ that synthesizes the electric with the magnetic ether to establish EMOTIONAL INTELLIGENCE...the heart. An aligned matrix establishes a super-human Emotional Intelligence that has 6 senses, instead of just 5 senses. Extra Sensory Perception (ESP) is the 6th sense that is the result of an aligned personality living within the parameters of the Laws of Nature. Many of us have moments of ESP awareness, just as many of us have moments that our heart's desire is manifest. The challenge is maintaining a consistent ability to manifest our heart's desire. It is the crushing inconsistency of our creative ability that forces us back into the disappointing realm of self-doubt and powerlessness; according to the *'Right Use of Will'*, this is called a *"reversal"* – a fall back into the ways of feeling impotent when it comes to creating what it is we desire to experience. This energetic conundrum is how a Light Body polarizes, creating an electromagnetic repulsion like the magnets that push one another apart = self-rejection.

The reciprocity or lack of reciprocity between the 4 parts of our personality determines whether or not we are capable of integrating the myriad points of view of our personality and, therefore, have the capacity to form an aligned decision about what we desire to experience. However, this cannot occur if the personality harbors a belief like "wanting it my way is selfish" or "attachment to outcome is wrong", etc. etc. etc. There are countless beliefs within the current paradigm that cancel out our ability to create what we desire, and they currently form a web of black magic that we are trapped within and trying to stay positive about.

If North and South are not in alignment, East and West experience disparity and war, such as the Battle of the Sexes. The East and West have been at war for some time now and we currently call it *'The War on Terror'*. With all due respect, waging war against Intimidating Form is like shooting oneself in the foot in order to stay safe! To understand how we continually create Intimidating Form, we must first understand our electromagnetic matrix that is our Light Body, as powered by the sun and earth and orchestrated by our unique heart.

The vibratory frequency of electric and magnetic ether has a wide array of sound that correlates with color, and, together, these forces of the metaphysical realm maintain a body of flesh and blood by maintaining a resonant frequency. Each of us forms a unique *Heart Song* of personality, but, unfortunately, we have been producing morbid songs of degeneration, estrangement and eventual death because of the universal spell we are under. I will say that there are some very nasty players out there, but I don't believe that they are reacting to anything other than our collective denial. Once we stop killing ourselves, and align ourselves to be pro-life, that type of intimidating form will go away. However, in the meantime, having orgasm under the influence of the Battle of the Sexes will only create more Intimidating Form! What basis do I have to say this? How is it we are creating abuse and war when our birthright is Free Will? I say this with compassion for the confusing ways we have been indoctrinated to deny our involvement in what many call "fate". The difference between *fate* and *Free Will* is as symbiotic as the yin/yang. As this principle begins to make more sense to you, it becomes easier to take the reigns of your unique intent and set this into form for no other reason than to please your heart.

What happens to the portals of the Light Body when we suppress our truth by pushing down our authentic emotional expression? Refusing magnetic essence entry to our heart prevents the magnetic ether from bonding with the electric ether in this citadel of exchange between East and West. This lack of reciprocity is crippling our ability to hold the silver ether present, as well, this electromagnetic repulsion leads to chronic loss of resonant frequency that robs us of the Will to live, leading only to death. For some, this is an agonizingly slow form of violence, while for others, it is abrupt ...overall, death is personal.

The *thought-forms* that stem from Death-Consciousness set off a domino of events that inevitably ends with the death of the body as predicted by the youthful heart. Ancient beliefs that have forever and a day been proven by our outer world, like: "no one gets out of this alive" or "death and taxes are the only certainty" or "everything in nature dies, and so will I" continue to hold us captive as a group. When we understand that everything does not die in nature, such as Microzyma and understand that the water in our body is responding to what we whole-heartedly believe in, then we may want to re-think our dominant paradigm. Especially, once we find out the special properties of the human heart. In fact, one of the MOST amazing aspects of the human heart is that it is NOT SUBJECT TO THE LAW'S OF ENTROPY (the Newtonian Principle that describes everything as subject to entropy, or falling apart and disintegrating with time). I will speak more about the heart's special properties in Chapter 5, for now I need to suggest new thought-forms that will help you begin the process that is Pangasm.

Here are a few new beliefs to replace the death-consciousness that was installed in our youth:

THE WILL TO LIVE IS A FORCE OF NATURE.

DESIRE IS THE ALCHEMY OF MAGIC.

PROVIDENCE IS LOVE AND MERCY IN NATURE.

THE BODY IS A MIRACLE OF OPPORTUNITY.

THE BODY HEALS ITSELF.

THE BODY WANTS TO LIVE.

ELECTROMAGNETIC ETHER IS AVAILABLE AT ALL TIMES FROM UP ABOVE AND DOWN BELOW.

MY SPECIAL HEART IS WHAT KEEPS ME IN LOVE.

THE DARKNESS HOLDS THE UNIVERSES TOGETHER.

DARK MATTER IS CONSCIOUS AND WANTS TO SUPPORT ME.

THE FEMININE DARK REALM IS A LOVING PRESENCE.

The way Pangasm begins to work magic in our heart is through choosing to adjust the belief patterns that have kept the emotional self in a relative prison of suppressed, oppressed, and compressed self-doubt that comes from feeling WRONG about our emotional truth... we are scared and trying not to notice. In fact, there is a cultural war targeting fear and making it the scapegoat of our chronic imbalance when it actually *IS* reasonable to be frightened of imbalance!

When chronic imbalance begins to show itself physically, we need to be aware that we are now in the critical stage of planning and implementing our death. Tracking emotional expressions about imbalance can give insight to our personal belief patterns so that one can release these beliefs, then solutions that lead to adaptation arise, rather than more devolutionary collapse! Releasing erroneous D-Con thought-forms is as easy as saying, "I no longer believe my body is unresponsive".

The basic difference between EVOLUTION AND DEVOLUTION, according to the Principle of Pangasm, lies within the cycles of Time and Space -- Evolution moves in elliptical cycles of perpetual motion forever and a day expanding and contracting like the breath you now inhale; however, within the cycles of death, devolution rules the day. Devolution is characterized by expansion and collapse, much the same way that a chronically acidic cell collapses and mutates into a morbid state. If the integrity of the life form cannot survive because of chronic stress, then nature moves to transform it through death, this is Mercy in action. Devolution is like the pendulum swinging between two polar extremes of itself, and eventually losing momentum until it is at a stand still. Evolution, on the other hand, moves in cycles of expansion & contraction and is potentially self-sustaining when the personality chooses life and adapts as a result.

In the past, the magnetic feminine principle of the Yin (the negative polarity) has been identified with the dark and unmoving presence of guilt to the point that it is currently difficult to tell the difference between the two. The nature of guilt is nothingness that is devoid of vibration and the end result of chronically harboring guilt is personality suicide. This is what chronic self-rejection in the form of silent shame/blame requires of life...personality suicide. Guilt lodges itself into our electromagnetic matrix, thereby, affecting all other physical systems by compelling the emotional ether to turn in on itself to establish devolution as the dominant paradigm. This *Unmitigated Duality* creates two separate hemispheres of personality that are not reciprocal; continually leading to the magnetic conundrum that is, once again, the Battle of the Sexes.

As a result of disengaging our emotions, the mind has been evolving itself through better thinking while the emotional self is cowering like a beaten dog. In this way, our emotional evolution comes to a screeching halt. The human condition has this ingenious mind dragging its child-like emotional self around and forcing it to perform like a trained dog...this is heartlessness!

Even though I tell you today that blame and shame are useless avenues of genuine resolution, it is essential that we create a safe place for the un-evolved emotional expressions of blaming-rage, abject terror and unremitting grief to speak their truth as a means of vibrating guilt out of our Light Body through sound and emotional movement. In this way, the portals of the Light Body get purged of the emotional congestion that had formed rigid magnetic blocks through chronically denying our truthful expression since childhood. This does not mean that we should hurl this denied negativity at others when it begins to move up to our heart for expression, however, sometimes it is difficult to hold this ethic if we have deeply denied our negativity for years or even decades.

Just what do I mean when I say "vibrating guilt out of the Light Body?" Often when we have strong emotions that we deem inappropriate, we try to choke them down and keep a straight face. While under the influence of alcohol or in later years this compressed emotional block jumps out of the confines of the mind's over-control and floods the room with, often, very embarrassing expressions. The game of *Pangasm* is a game that is designed to help us get this magnetic congestion moving within an atmosphere of acceptance for the disturbance, rather than yet more shame and the ensuing self-rejection that comes from feeling wrong about our core truth. It is possible to move emotions without the game, since these denied emotions will not stay in a state of denial indefinitely and under pressure they often blow like an emotional volcano.

Living around others that share the ethic of *Pangasm* creates a relatively safe place for the balancing process of emotional movement to vibrate the negativity it was forced to deny in the past. In this way, we can magnetically align North and South to become reciprocal once again while sharing intimately with others. This is much better than going through this process alone. Sometimes the purging of the emotional self can be quite interesting, and, if kept in perspective, can create endless laughter and camaraderie. Even so, without honesty healing does not occur.

It is not possible to purge the energetic blocks in our Light Body with thought alone. This is where the 'positive thinking' crowd loses ground to random and inconsistent results. Holding back our authentic truth is like jamming an electrical circuit and shorting it out. When our emotions are suppressed and the vibration of our truth becomes stagnant in the darkness of guilt, our magnetic field loses impetus and stops moving...we call this depression. No amount of drugs or positive thinking will change this problem. The emotional intensity of vibration that was initially suppressed needs to be expressed in order for that which was denied to move through the matrix, purging it of the nothingness (guilt) that was given to the heart in exchange for our truth. We do not have to wait for the emotions to move on their own (especially if the emotional self is in a clinch of death and unmoving) because this therapeutic game is a great way to bring it all out of the closet in a very dynamic and intimate way, sooner than later; as a result, you will definitely begin feeling again.

The Principle of Pangasm offers the *LANGUAGE OF SHAMELESSNESS* with the understanding that "right" and "wrong", or "good" and "bad" are the expression of the extremes of imbalance or the extremes of devolution. Once we take the value judgments of shame and blame out of the conversation, then we witness that there is simply BALANCE OR IMBALANCE. Having said that, those who consciously choose to over-ride the Will of another personality will harbor guilt, as it should be! Because, this over-riding becomes arrested by the presence of guilt, unless an individual is a socio-path, (incapable of feeling remorse, guilt or much of anything.) This principle does not address this peculiar human problem (that of a sociopath) and is only concerned with the souls who still have an emotional ability to feel and the personal integrity that desires no harm upon the other.

Accepting chronic imbalance as normal is a misunderstanding that is rooted in the age-old Battle of the Sexes and invariably leads to violence. Whether that is violence against others or self-destructiveness depends upon the Original Cause of the individual or group. Whatever type of erroneous thought-forms that led to the imbalance is the source of our Original Cause. Many children on earth are preyed upon sexually and are further damaged by the stigma associated with this pattern, causing a domino of emotional, mental and physical problems that pervade modern societies. In fact, sexual abuse is a long-reaching problem in our societies and has been effectually covered-up by the denial of complicit adults, including religious leaders who claim to represent God, yet deny corruption within their own ranks. Fortunately, we live in a time when technology is exposing the worst of the worst realities the earth has chosen to hold presence for, while she maintained an ever-loving vigil to provide a climatic status quo for us to eventually evolve the type of integrity that is founded upon love for self and the other.

The game of *Pangasm* always leads a pair to revisit any sexual shame that is lodged in our matrix of electromagnetic exchange and can make recovery from sexual abuse a feasible possibility, rather than spending a life-time coping with an emotional body that is within the clinch of deep shame.

Attending to the mental plane while rejecting the emotional aspect of our self will definitely kill the Will to live and explains why some prayers work and others do not. If there is denial/guilt that is blocking reciprocity between the 4 parts, the prayer is not grounded in reality, but is, instead, a mental exercise. Creating an aligned agreement field, in regard to our heart's desire, is the way to create balance, abundance and satisfaction. However, providence does not appreciate giving freely only to stand by and witness the body get demonized as unresponsive, when in fact, it is magically responsive! Our body is only able to be responsive to our desire for it to maintain health and beauty as long as we are not killing it with denial. Denied negativity shreds a Light Body. We cannot deny the truth about the Laws of Nature and expect to create a reality we actually enjoy from our denial. Although we have gotten away with this seemingly forever, the earth has simply had enough...especially now that every nation insists upon developing nuclear warheads that could seriously puncture the earth's delicate atmosphere. The plants and animals that are evolving on earth deserve her consideration, as well.

The Battle of the Sexes leads to a 3-dimensional, linear reality that is evil (evil is the word LIVE spelled backwards and it is the word I use to describe Devolution - suggesting that the evildoer has given up on life at a fundamentally vital level). Devolution is linear, and, therefore, devoid of any kind of sustainability for lack of reciprocity, which is why *HEARTLESSNESS* is the human condition. If, however, the intellect is in alignment with the emotional self, then the heart of Love is born from self-acceptance. Only self-love will allow for the ETHER OF LOVE to hold space open in our Heart, thereby, making the body real through maintaining a vital resonant frequency. This is the alchemy of magic and is like having a GENII IN A BOTTLE that is capable of offering limitless experience in a physical body that has the potential to make our every wish come true (unless one wants to harm self or others).

Heartlessness is the current Human Condition and it has crippled civilization, to the point that we collectively believe that humankind is evil. This collective judgment renders all, who adopt this thought-form, to harbor guilt to the point of eventually becoming so guilt-ridden that they lose the ability to be honest and trust others. This is the '*Original Sin*' of shame that constitutes a deadly form of self-rejection. This poison estranges young and old without prejudice. The guilt that comes from overriding or manipulating others can never be resolved unless the overriding of others stops, because guilt is meant to immobilize those who practice injustice...this is *JUSTICE*. These checks and balances are beautifully demonstrated by the elements of life.

As I stated before, humanity is holding a devolving, destructive position because of our collective paradigm. The collective consciousness of humanity not only denies life emotionally, it also denies life physically. This is the basis of self-rejection, leading to shame and body hatred most of which is being held in a volatile state of denial. When we come into balance by integrating the parts of our personality, ether stays present to help us live indefinitely in a manifest body of flesh and blood comprised of immortal particles and responsive water that issue a holographic maze powered by the sun and earth. Our emotions are the motor that keeps our hologram humming with magnetic life force, helping our heart to beat the rhythm of a unique personality that is filled with the Light of Love.

During times of orgasm, ether moves through our Light Body as a quantum force. If the matrix of our Light Body is blocked in anyway, the orgasmic flow of ether will threaten our very life. This is why teens have such a high rate of suicide compared to the rest of our society. Upon the first orgasm, deeply ingrained beliefs about reality get a surge of ether that threatens our truth if that truth is founded upon the Battle of the Sexes and powered by a death-urge surge of ether!

The collective emotional body of humanity is currently in dire circumstances because of the repetitive patterns of estrangement and death that are being passed off as normal and balanced, even being called "Gods Will for us"! When the emotional self is forced to stay quiet about this ghoulish anti-life, endless violence plagues our every turn as religious ideals try to convince us that we are heroes for our suffering somehow while we faithfully wait to go to a better place. This is the cycle of hopelessness that is willing to suffer chronic imbalance for some promise of a better future. As a result of the hopelessness that we have developed, regarding the life and death cycle, we have demonized the negative emotional warning system that is designed to alert us about the misunderstanding that perpetuates this cycle of imbalance. As a result, we all seem to be waiting in some lackluster reality that never seems to deliver the goods, so to speak.

The earth is the source of our *Golden Ether* -- it is this magnetic essence that draws that which we desire to us constituting the basis of human magnetism. However, if we are in denial of our desire, because of false ideas about the wicked nature of desire, we will draw any number of experiences, because we have successfully disengaged the Will by adopting thought-forms that limit our personal sovereignty. As a result, we lose our way because we no longer trust the human Will to be appropriate or to deliver what it is we desire. This is the nasty aspect of Devolution, as this insidious misunderstanding leads us to believe in right vs. wrong and good vs. evil. If we take the value judgment out of our experience, we find there is simply positive, neutral and negative. The neutral part is our heart and it can and will hold a perfect balance between our positive and negative polarity if we are not in rejection of our negative polarity, which is the **Feminine Principle of Darkness**...the YIN.

Instead of judging anything or person as "right" or "wrong", "good" or "bad", we can begin to witness balance and imbalance as the variable. In this way, we can disengage from judging reality from the shame/blame position of guilt and stop creating 'Human Garbage' through acting out our dehumanizing paradigm. As we remove value judgments from our heart through judgment release using our word, we can begin to comfortably express our current imbalance without being made wrong for having imbalance. In this way, the path will open for us to express the imbalance and evolve through self-acceptance capable of comprehending a pro-life paradigm. (Note: I do not use the term "pro-life" to align this message with the current controversies about birth-control issues).

Just as the rainbow has a full spectrum of primary and secondary colors, the human emotional self has a full spectrum of positive and negative emotions. The negative emotions of fear, anger and sadness (among others) have been the scapegoat for their attempts to warn us of the long-running imbalance caused by the human paradigm. If we disable the warning system that is our negative emotions, we lose the ability to feel the truth, and, thereby, lose the ability to prevent the domino of disaster that comes from calling chronic imbalance normal or beyond our influence.

Let me get a little redundant here, please. If you remember anything from my words at all let it be about the sorry, sorry state of the individual and collective emotional body on earth today. Children and psychic adults are the first to feel the pressure of collective denial. Unfortunately, for most psychics, trying to make sense of the Battle of the Sexes within their own inner plane is paradoxical at best and painful to be certain. One of the unfortunate results of this pattern today is that children in the US are being drugged, en masse, as they witness a War on Drugs!

The misunderstanding that stems from living our lives as if we do not have a choice about whether our body is healthy, or not, has far reaching ramifications that devastate well-meaning people by leading them to eventually lose the Will to live with endless oppression, violence and debilitation that they truly believe they have no power to affect in meaningful ways. Our very own Genii dwells in and around our body and wants to provide us with our heart's desire. Once we stop denying our emotional truth, we will be able to create balance and access our birthright. This game is designed to reconnect our electromagnetic field in a way that gives us access to the divine gift that a human heart is.

Creation is perpetually knocking on our door of perception to offer options for life everlasting, yet, we were taught to deny this part of ourselves to the point of losing vibration that does not have the ability to sustain physical existence. We are not wrong for adopting denial because we have all been enacting a gross misunderstanding in the name of Love for eons. However, if we refuse the balancing potential that the truth is attempting to illustrate for us in this moment, we will certainly go the way of the silent majority who firmly believe that they have no choice about how their body responds or does not respond.

Vibratory, magnetic ether is the vital life force that most people are searching for and it is available at all times from the ground under our feet. It has been forced to create hell on earth in the name of love through orgasm that is shared in the presence of guilt. When guilt silently lives in our heart, it pervades our nervous system and tortures those who love us. Self-doubt creates shame by putting into place an anti-dynamic, magnetic rejection of self. Undoing the black magic of indoctrinated self-rejection by triggering a sexual response capable of rendering our crown and root as open and reciprocal is unpredictably dynamic, and it is within this moment of true openness that we can adopt the self-concept that best fits our heart and effectually release self from the bonds of linear existence while having intimacy with the other.

When some of the participants of an imbalanced situation take responsibility while others do not, then denial is present. This is the trap of a linear, un-reciprocal reality that demonizes others as a means of attempting to creating balance. Our society would look and function much differently if True Free Will had designed its institutions and traditions. Having said that, I do not presently believe that we must collapse this society in order to begin anew. The limits inherent in the Battle of the Sexes will mutate quite rapidly when just two people hold an agreement to choose life everlasting. Consider it done.

OVERVIEW OF CHAPTER FOUR:

1. Golden magnetic Ether is available at all times from the earth. Silver electric Ether is available from the sun at all times, but cannot be held present in our Light Body unless the magnetic Ether is allowed up into our heart as EMOTIONAL INTELLIGENCE.

2. The willingness to express a full spectrum of negative and positive human emotion is what draws the magnetic ETHER up into our heart for our unique expression as the essential motion of maintaining a RESONANT FREQUENCY.

3. Thought-forms based upon misunderstanding about the nature of the negative polarity motivate a soul to suppress emotion. By releasing judgments that deny the Laws of Nature, we become open to custom-made solutions and opportunities we did not previously consider.

4. The universal indoctrination process that occurs to all humans forces the masses into denying their survival terror in a way that produces constant INTIMIDATING FORM.

5. Allowing magnetic Ether to move into our heart as emotional expression is the exchange that enables a human Light Body to behave as our personal *Genii in a Bottle* by drawing to us what it is we desire to experience, rather than continual intimidating form that is capable of exhausting our Will

CHAPTER 5

ELEMENT AIR

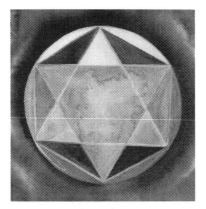

HEARTSONG

Molecular oxygen is one of the most important substances on earth. Oxygen comprises 21% of the atmosphere, 89% of seawater by weight, and at least 47% of the Earth's crust. Almost all living organisms utilize oxygen for energy generation and respiration. In the 1840's, Michael Faraday discovered that oxygen is attracted to a magnet. When our blood is low in iron, as in Anemia, we are less able to bond oxygen with our hemoglobin (blood). Here we can see that oxygen is responsive to consciousness, because it is the consciousness that must choose to take action to provide for the body's needs, such as securing nutrition that will enable the body to maintain health. Just as dust particles respond to our cellular pH by creating cellular health or morbidity, oxygen also chemically responds to a person's ability/inability or desire/lack of desire, to maintain good physical health. According to the World Hunger Education Service, over two billion people, approximately 30% of the worlds' population, are anemic and in many cases are subject to a larger population that has not established sustainability.

A portion of Gaia's inhabitants are getting their own basic needs met while a substantial portion of the population is not. The injustice of resource distribution that allows disparity of this proportion is apparently corrupt, as the upper class looks out upon the sea of despairing humanity and blames the poor for their plight...just like the emotions are getting blamed for reflecting the imbalance created by the Battle of the Sexes. Those that have legislated the laws for the many have created an atmosphere of derision toward anyone who wants to be negative about the status quo while at the same time have confused the public by calling corruption 'leadership'. There is no one to blame for this reflection, as the elected officials are educating the masses about the corrupt dominant paradigm that has laid a faulty foundation complete with perverse god-concepts, worldwide hunger and dis*EASE*.

The lack of willingness to take responsibility for the poverty among us is another example of how those who are polarized to positive/positive are treating their own negative polarity... their emotional body. The poor and sick among us represent the effect that the collective paradigm has upon the collective body of mankind. This is the denied state that our collective emotional body finds itself in today...starving for sustenance, attention and understanding. In other words desperate!

Releasing beliefs that were put into place eons ago is like reprogramming a computer. It is possible to do this now, because during this epic of the human adventure, we are being taken (by means of the communication revolution, and an Astronomical-cycle that has the earth embroiled in a planetary Melt-water) back to the beginning of time when we created the paradigm that humanity currently operates within. Many of the ancient Shaman religions recognize this current epoch as cosmically linked to our astronomical relationship with our galaxy and larger universe. Religion is helping us to realize the belief structures that created the current reality we suffer from and science is helping us to recognize how we devolved to this place.

The ancient Maya demonstrated precise astronomical calculations and their knowledge of human energetic systems rivals the modern scientific understandings about topics such as humanity's genetic code. As well, modern science is helping us to understand our biological capacity in a way that demonstrates that we are only playing with 20 cards in a deck of 64.

DNA is our personal blueprint and, as such, contains all our mental, physical, emotional and spiritual information. The DNA holds within its memory the blueprint of who we are physically, such as the color of our hair and eyes, and even the tendency for risk-taking, shyness and hereditary illnesses. The DNA strand has a possible 64 Codons, and at this time on earth, most people are only accessing 20 to 24 Codon levels (*'The Sacred Flower of Life – Part II'* by, Drunvalo Melchizedek). This limitation is one of the reasons why most all of humanity is only able to comprehend the linear realm of the 3rd dimension and why only a small portion of our brain is utilized at this time. Truly, mankind has bio-spiritual potential that is waiting idly by for our summons.

The human genome is a universe in and of itself and each of us has access to the software of personality. One of the reasons we are accessing only a small part of our brain is because the human condition continually guides a soul to deplete their magnetic field by denying their F.E.A.R (false-evidence-appearing-real). This disassociation from authentic emotional truth eventually robs one of the Will to move as they descend into the self-limiting pit of devolution.

It has been scientifically proven that memory improves when the emotions are involved.[4] Therefore, it is reasonable to suggest

---

4   "Some theorists believe that a small lump of brain tissue, a portion of the limbic system known as the hippocampus, plays the part of a "record" button, much like the button you press on a tape recorder to make it record what you say into the microphone. The hippocampus, which

that emotional connection to experience indelibly imprints the experience into our personality for permanent record. Without emotional connection, the experience is similar to a fleeting thought that is not grounded in the emotional root to become a part of our personality.

When the magnetic polarity is in alignment with the electric polarity, the heart of love is born (self-acceptance that refuses to harm self and the other) and the body becomes real. Becoming energetically sustainable means maintaining a viable resonant frequency that establishes a personality grounded in the root and reciprocal in the heart with our crown. For those who remain in electromagnetic reversal (when our root and crown are in magnetic repulsion), their resonant frequency will continue to decline to effectually disassociate the personality from reality, to the point that the laws of nature will relieve him or her of having to suffer the ravages of chronic stress through death. Whereas, it is the intent of the *Principle of Pangasm* to alert people to the fact that this is a choice we face, not necessarily an act of fate or biology that is beyond our control.

Even if you do not whole-heartedly believe in a personal God, I would bet you at least believe in Love. When our heart is actively engaged in its own existence through the power of Emotional Intelligence, we begin to operate within the 4th dimension of personal divinity that is steeped within the Light of unconditional love. How would I define unconditional Love? It is the act of loving one's self enough to

---

also has a variety of other functions, seems to respond to the general emotional level you experience at any one instant. This theory holds that if your brain is not particularly aroused, either because you are not paying attention or because you are not very interested in what you are perceiving, or both, the hippocampus tends to have less influence over the transfer of the images of short-term processing to long-term storage. But if you find the scene, object, or idea somewhat engrossing, or if you become more aroused as a result of your recognition of its meaning, the hippocampus presumably sends more and stronger "record" signals to whatever neural structures carry out the long-term imprinting process. *'Brain Power: Learn to Improve Your Thinking Skills', by Karl Albrecht – pg 265-66*

speak one's whole-hearted truth at all times. This is tricky, as denial has within it, built in blind spots that serve to keep us doubting our own truth. This is why this game is dedicated to enabling the participants to stimulate the magnetic field to move up the channel to their heart for expression of what was denied, thereby making the rigid magnetic matrix (that was previously in repel between the crown and root) to liquefy and mutate into a reciprocal exchange that opens space for the participants to bond within the sanctuary of self-acceptance and trust.

The important aspect that establishes the game of *Pangasm* as a therapeutic technique is that it increases the chances that we will receive understanding rather than more judgment that could send one into a spiral of confusion and self-doubt. By simply feeling accepted by the other, we increase our white blood count and enhance our immune system, not to mention opening the way for genuine friendship and possibly romantic ties that are founded upon honesty.

Ultimately, whether or not we ever come out of our self-made closet of estrangement of shame and blame, the truth is that we will never be able to trick our self into creating balance through continued self-rejection (withholding our truth in a state of silent shame). When all is said and done, the only soul we are tricking when we consciously choose to subvert our truth is our own unique heart that depends upon our consciousness accepting our emotional truth over the illusion of a presentation of balance. *This is the ultimate spiritual decision that we face on a daily basis.*

The heart and lungs feed the body with blood and oxygen in a sublime co-operative function. The human heart contains specialized cells that are 4th dimensional and in a dimension that's difficult for mortals to access because they are steeped in Death Consciousness. In a State of Grace (the unified 9th dimension), the human heart holds our North, South, East and West together with the electromagnetic harmony of love when in alignment with the 5 elements. Thanks to science we are now able to measure and better understand the human electromagnetic field generated by our unique heart rhythm, blood content and flow, as well as, a highly charged neurological network.

Recently, studies have shown that the heart muscle is able to interact energetically with other hearts that are not sharing the same physical location. Through the study of heart transplant patients, much has come to light about the special properties of the human heart. In his book, *The Heart's Code*, the Hawaiian heart surgeon, Dr. Paul Pearsall, codified the special characteristics of the human heart. He identifies the special electromagnetic energy that the heart conducts as "L" energy and describes how this Life Force operates. "Heart cells also communicate bio-chemically, but unlike brain or any other body cells, they also seem able to exchange life information by using a subtle and as yet immeasurable vital force." He goes on to say, "The heart is uniquely composed of 'L' energy… The heart's EMF [electromagnetic field] is five thousand times more powerful than the electromagnetic field created by the brain and, in addition to its immense power, has subtle, non-local effects that travel within these forms of energy."

What I find to be the most relevant and fascinating aspect revealed by Dr. Pearsall's studies is that the human heart is not subject to entropy. Even "L" energy does not seem to diminish over time while all of the other known forms of energy seem to follow most of the Newtonian laws of physics. This special electromagnetic field of the human heart seems to be the glue, the actual stuff, of the extraordinary sentiment known as love.

When I read The Heart's Code, I was so incredibly moved to learn the special properties of my heart and I was relieved that scientists were proving that the metaphysical world is perfectly aligned with the biological world. In our special and unique heart rests the capacity of a personality to unite heaven and earth in our body. Just as the building blocks of all blood, plant and tissue (Microzyma) on earth are not subject to entropy and never die, so is the heart muscle potentially immortal.

Even though the heart's energy is subtle, its physical manifestations are powerful, unlike any other muscle in the body and unless it is afflicted with disease, the heart muscle does not seem to weaken with age. This metaphysical organ is never still, even if a patient is declared "brain dead" the heart can continue to beat on its own. Through a process no scientists can fully explain, a heart removed from its body still remembers how to beat, sometimes for several minutes.

"The heart beats approximately one hundred thousand times a day and forty million times a year. For more than seventy years, it supplies the pumping capacity for nearly three billion cardiac pulsations and propels more than two gallons of blood per minute through the body. The heart transports about one hundred gallons of blood per hour through a vascular system that, if extended, could be wrapped around the earth two and one half times and each fiber of that system is crammed full of the info-energy traveling through it, helping that 'L' energy to broadcast energy everywhere like a huge vascular antenna" (*The Heart's Code,* Pearsall).

As a result of spending his entire life codifying the special properties of the human heart, Dr. Pearsall comfortably reports that there is a high probability that a heart transplant patient will automatically acquire personality traits that belonged to the heart donor. Through this information I was able to understand that the heart is the seat of our soul and has the ability to influence all other organs of our body, especially if the personality has embraced Emotional Intelligence as a lifestyle. Furthermore, this fascinating work has revealed that the human heart is the organ that has, within its cellular structure, memory of emotional intelligence that is transported with our personality from life-time to life-time. In essence, our heart muscle is a cellular memory bank of all our past lives!

"A mind out of touch with its own heart joins into a lethal alliance with its body."

This last statement by Dr. Pearsall describes Death Consciousness in a nutshell! When imbalance reaches a chronic state we polarize to one end of our spectrum or another, rather than being HEART CENTERED. When the emotional intelligence of the heart is constantly over-ridden by the brain because the emotions have been judged as "inappropriate", "illogical", "selfish" or "disturbing", we begin to climb into the lonely tower of self, which is actually a vacuum of self. This is the place where intimacy goes to die and the place where secrets form to estrange us from others. We have been very creative in dressing up this cage with common beliefs such as, "secrets make people more interesting", "showing our authentic interest in a potential mate will make us boring, less desirable" or "playing hard to get will keep the other interested in me". Truly, we have tried to make heartlessness an acceptable state of being.

Whether from blame or shame, the estrangement process of a frightened mind brings about the same result...devolution. When the mind attempts to inform the emotional self what its emotional response should be, the mind is robbing us of the root's ability to establish emotional intelligence. In a state of balance, the mind performs the interpretive function not the selective function, however, when the mind steps in to inform the emotional body about how it should feel, the pattern becomes that of devolution and closely replicates the collapse of a cell in a chronic acidic state or the collapse of an entire civilization.

Devolution, if left unchecked, always collapses the human coil by destroying the reciprocity between the Crown and the Root in the heart. This is how we polarize to either negative/negative or positive/positive patterns of imbalance. This is the moment ugliness begins to ride the soul into the sanctuary of death.

When we separate ourselves from others through secrets and lies and rely upon our mind to tell us what is true, we live in a vacuum of self that refuses to learn from others, refuses to commune with others intimately while ceasing to vibrate electromagnetic ether into a state of alignment with the other. Having relations with other hearts is the means by which we evolve through experience. If we have thought-forms that close us off from vibratory interactions with others, we begin a slow form of devolution that springs from the hopelessness of heartlessness.

Acute heartlessness is devoid of emotional vibration.

The mortal Light Body is linear because it is not reciprocal (freely exchanging electromagnetic properties), therefore, it is hemorrhaging its ether on a continual basis making it impossible for the heart to maintain integrity between the upper and lower worlds. In other words, our heart cannot hold the parts of self together if death is embraced and installed into our heart. This pattern always collapses the mortal coil of the individual because they are praying for death subconsciously on a daily basis through their pervasive belief in the inevitability of death. Hence, the mortal death wish that comes from being indoctrinated into the Battle of the Sexes. If we hold death in our heart as our future transformative event, then that is exactly what we will get because True Free Will is the way in which the Laws of Nature deliver justice to a personality through evolution.

Our Root (body) has a different nature than our Crown (brain), yet has forever been told by the intellect that there was something evil or deficient about the nature of our emotional body and the nature of our physical body, leading humanity to use the mind to over-ride emotion and universally view the body as disposable, not to mention disgusting. These judgments are energetic thought-forms that create magnetic blocks, eventually causing physical systems to begin collapsing as the result of this perverse form of self-rejection.

The parts of self have consciousness and are responding to our paradigm by creating it. The body is terribly distressed to have to perform this service for the delusional personality, explaining why the Battle of the Sexes is often called, "the Body/Spirit Split" by many esoteric scholars. The body has been rebelling against the personality by trying to stay alive. Within this paradoxical paradigm the emotional body is stuck between these points of view desperately attempting to appease both sides while the Heart is lost. Hence, "Universal Heartlessness" is being called normal.

Collectively denied hopelessness has brought about judgment fields that suggest, "to identify the problem is the same as creating the problem", when, the actual truth is: if the problem is not identified, the imbalance cannot be evolved into a state of balance through communication, reciprocation, understanding and action.

Negative judgments about the dark ether that spirals up from the earth are partially the result of our collective confusion about guilt. Guilt is the by-product of the persistent rejection of our individual emotional truth and is a different kind of darkness than the feminine polarity's magnetic darkness of EMOTIONAL ETHER. When the mind refuses our emotional truth, guilt (which is nothingness that does not vibrate) enters our heart, takes the place of our vital electromagnetic ether, and the exchange systems become blocked causing unmitigated duality.

BECAUSE OF THE CONFUSION ABOUT THE NEGATIVE POLARITY OF DARKNESS, SELF-DOUBT HAS TAKEN THE PLACE OF SELF-ACCEPTANCE, EFFECTIVELY KEEPING CHRONIC IMBALANCE THE NORM.

The energetic blocks in our Light Body correlate with physical blocks and vise versa. Within the paradigm of death, our Light Body and Physical Body lack the integrity to hold self together and are demonstrating this on a constant basis as debilitation and death. When we are energetically un-reciprocal, our elemental body dutifully begins a gradual decomposition of self due to a descending vibratory field.

In regard to entropy, the heart is capable of giving an aligned personality the capacity to boost into a unified dimension where our word becomes physical reality. In other words, we develop the ability to manifest our desire from the breath of life that speaks as a unified personal prayer, establishing a sacred moment where the personality wields the stuff of magic.

Most of us were reciprocal before we learned about death and before we formed our current self-concept. In essence, we need to go back to the pre-personal stage and rewire our matrix. Because of the timing of this disconnect, we have lost the memory that would help us understand our own individual responsibility for choosing this disconnect. This is why the solutions of blame and shame have been the avenues of descent that forced us to live in "Hell on Earth" and terminal estrangement!

True self-acceptance leads to a form of shamelessness that is about understanding our sexual essence as a force to be expressed with dignity. Guilt has forced us to view the blessing of sexual desire as a problem to be controlled. However, suppressing the truth about our sexual expression comes from feeling wrong about our desire and eons of this insane sexual ethic has perverted the divine gift, that sex is, into dark and terrible expressions that over-ride others, such as sexual slavery and pedophilia.

When I became aware of how immense the denied guilt was in my own body, I became suicidal for the first time in my life after the age of 40. Thank goodness I told loved ones what I was going through so that this insane drive did not fester within a vacuum of guilt long enough to lead me to lose the Will to live entirely. When we block the reciprocity of ether through adopting guilt, we lose the Will to move. Many people call this symptom laziness, which is just another way of rejecting the truth that we just want to lie down and die already!

If we wish to stay present for the resolution occurring upon Gaia, then it is important that we dissolve the guilt that is keeping our metaphysical Light Body from being reciprocal. Simply wishing for this and sprinkling Fairy dust will certainly disappoint the ardent New Age soul, however, understanding the mechanism of the human Light Body and, thereby, activating it, will deliver a very satisfying response. I know of this first hand and continue to benefit from this simple information in fulfilling and interesting ways, even though I still suffer from various forms of denial, as indicated by my own form.

Unfortunately, we cannot clear unmoving guilt out of our matrix through positive thinking alone because the congestion is magnetic and the thinking part of us is not the magnetic aspect that has the blocks. Only emotional vibration can recalibrate a stuck matrix. Of course, the beliefs need to be identified and adjusted in order to effectively choose life, however, simply changing our mind does not address the stuck and unmoving magnetic matrix that has been disrupted since childhood. The magnetic blocks that come from guilt can only be cleared through recreating the same vibratory intensity of the denied expression that guilt had originally blocked. Once we reach this emotional intensity, rigid magnetic patterns reform to allow for the new ideas of the evolving self-concept to open the way for electromagnetic reciprocity to become the new status quo.

The game of Pangasm is an effective way to access the magnetic part of self without having to intellectualize the process. It is much more rapid to have another who is willing to express within an intimate setting, where the two players can get to the core of the problem without feeling wrong for having disturbance. Truly, expressing our denied emotions in the presence of another who has acceptance for us is as important as expressing the denied emotions and releasing the judgments that keep the emotional pattern stuck. Being witnessed by a compassionate other is a very dynamic process that the game of Pangasm opens space for.

The common myth claiming that, "the ego is selfish" is a judgment within the disconnected mind that is desperately trying to control its body, its emotions and the world at large because control is considered necessary for survival.

Somewhere between the extreme poles of selflessness and selfishness is our unique balance-point of effortless existence.

The self-doubt that arises from denying that death has the ego backed into a corner creates a paranoid persona of self-rejection that must work overtime to present balance, when actually imbalance is crushing the heart's Will to Live! Establishing balance between the four parts of our personality will ultimately lead to balanced experiences and interactions with the outer world. Essentially, balance is an inside job that requires the soul to remain open to new or even "seemingly" miraculous solutions.

Within the context of the Battle of the Sexes, the dynamic characteristics of an evolutionary heart become static and unmoving, thereby, forcing the ego to attempt to manipulate the outer world in order to get desires met, because the inner world is lost in the collapsing spiral of the death grip. This is how we devolve into energetic vampires. However, taking responsibility for our energetic presence leads to identifying one's personal contribution to the problem of universal heartlessness. However, there is no resolution if there is no agreement that there is a problem, therefore, no understanding or adaptive action can evolve that is capable of changing the pattern of devolution, unless each participant is willing to take responsibility by becoming honest with their own self about their own distinct patterns of imbalance.

A magnetic field that has received decades of rejection is in a serious predicament if the blocks do not get addressed. Once emotional congestion reaches a chronic state, our physical and mental health declines and denied desperation begins to twist our features. On top of that, orgasm delivers an exponential amount of ether into our blocked matrix and will apply a dangerous level of pressure that threatens to manifest our currently held death wish. If orgasm is experienced in the presence of guilt, it can kill us sooner than we were planning. This is why millions of people find themselves in a chronic state of depression. It is in this stagnant environment that we currently find ourselves wondering whom to blame or feeling crushing levels of shame —usually both. The inner conversation of this dilemma is persistently about justifying our point of view because we are ashamed of what we have created. We are not wrong for getting stuck within the confines of this war, however, we cannot afford to continue to contribute to this suicidal death wish of the group, if, in fact, one is pro-life.

Depression is a temporary condition that is the result of a disabled magnetic field. Depression is a healthy response to our reality today because it is not a sign of good health to be well-adjusted to a sick society. To believe that our heart's desire is wrong, dirty, selfish or unrealistic will definitely lead one to feel uninspired, depressed and eventually ready to die! This state of existence is all too common and, for the most part, the agreement is to avoid addressing these confusing issues in favor of distractions and in favor of dismissing these patterns as unavoidable facts of life. Honestly, this problem will be quite simple to resolve once the collective begins to understand the Laws of Nature and realizes how to align the parts of personality with these providential laws. We are in alignment with the laws of nature, in that we persistently create estrangement, war and death from our collective paradigm; having said that, I imagine that most all people would choose intimacy, health and life if they knew they had a choice.

The magnetic ether of the yin is only dark when it is separate from its power source...the light of the yang. Separating the yin from the yang is horribly painful for the yin and leaves the yang without the ground under its feet. This separation makes the electric/masculine pole a disconnected sophistry (sophistry is a mental concept that is not grounded in physical reality) and forces the magnetic feminine pole to become erratic and desperate. Without the electric ether, the magnetic ether begins to lose vibration. If the magnetic vortex becomes stagnant because it is separate from its power source, it becomes more and more difficult for the emotional body to rise up into the heart in order to establish emotional intelligence. Many become so desensitized from their emotional body that they turn to violence and sexual perversity in an attempt to stimulate the emotional body to respond. Without the grounding affect of the yin, the yang cannot fully manifest in the physical plane, which then causes competition and strife between the East and West (Left and Right). These realities are punctuated by inequitable class systems, rape, famine, corruption and endless sacrifice in the name of an illusionary reality.

The song that naturally springs from reciprocity between the Crown and the Root is our special tune that expresses our commitment to truth or denial of it. Our Word is what the outer world hears while our heartbeat is the sound our inner world generates for the Universe to register our existence within the cosmic heartbeat of Providence. Instead of songs of wonder and love, mankind has been singing a long and drawn out Lament.

Why is it we continually use Providence to create brutality? The war against the dark principle of the Divine Miss Yin was demonstrated in the Dark Ages as the Catholic Church's 'European Inquisition'. This event was a violent, systematic purging of the matriarchy (feminine power structure) and is ironically called the "Dark Ages." During the matriarchal times healers were women and family names followed the mother's family name, however, the emerging masculine power structure of the church was in conflict with Pagan Earth Magic ways. This was largely because the church was trying to control the sexual practices of humanity through the use of guilt and violence as a resolution for a problem that had not yet been identified through Pagan practices and traditions. The church eliminated the practitioners of the feminine Pagan healing arts much like the mind of a person under the influence of D-Con perpetually over-rides the function of its emotional self as a way of taking control. I call this form of self-doubt 'discipline'. When we force discipline upon the realm of the feminine magnetic polarity (both genders have a male and female polarity), we stifle its natural flow, essentially separating its parts and ending movement...also known as laziness, frigidity, insanity, depression, etc.

One of the hallmarks of discipline is the collective judgment that believes: "If I act as I desire, I will surely lose control and harm myself or others".

IT IS IN THIS ENVIRONMENT THAT GOOD LITTLE GIRLS AND BOYS CRUCIFY THEIR DESIRE BODIES!

The current dominant paradigm of Patriarchy imposes a standard that establishes guilt as an authority about life as priests of the

Catholic Church have so painfully demonstrated for centuries! The perversion that replaces life-affirming consensual sex with abstinence that is enforced by guilt often manifests perverse patterns of behavior. Rather than maintain church-wide sexual abstinence among clergy, these types of religious decrees demonize the freedom of consensual sexual expression, which is a deadly projection of denied guilt, while carrying on institutionalized pedophilia.

Contrary to what most world religions teach, I want you to understand the life-force value of your orgasmic ether so that no person or group calling itself an authority can take your essence from you, if you do not want them to. Once you know what you actually have available to you, I am almost certain you will not wish to give it up or have others take it from you for any reason! Having said this, the church is not wrong for trying to control mankind's sexual expression because sex in the presence of guilt is creating perversion, estrangement and war. Now that we can look back on this sorry historical event, we can evolve by understanding that suppression, oppression, and persecution will not heal the problem of heartless sex.

During the European Inquisition, Catholic priests tortured and killed millions of European women and men in the name of an angry and jealous god. The official reason for this event was based upon the biblical story of Adam and Eve and the church's position that Eve was responsible for mankind falling from god's grace because of a snake, an apple and sexual shame. As a result of this misunderstanding, strict limits have been put into place against women and sexuality to this very day. This is the ghoulish reflection that raises guilt up while casting women down into a form of slavery and punishment that mimics the imbalance between the male and female that is reflecting the imbalance between the mind and its emotional body...Heaven and Earth.

Recently in Romania, (2005), a priest ordered nuns to crucify a young woman named Maricica Irina Cornici. She died alone in a cold, dark room after three days of being chained to a cross with no food or water and a towel shoved into her mouth. This is symbolic of the way we all attempt to silence the truthful expression about imbalance. The man who ordered this "exorcism" was a principle monk named Daniel Petru Corogeanu. Father Daniel probably considers himself an altruistic servant of God, however, he is standing in an ancient position of power that is enforcing the laws of a horrible misunderstanding! This is one reason why my heart is broken and why I am desperate to put my words into form as a warning to ALL who override the Will of others, especially in the name of God!

Mysticism and religion are in the same category with one another because, neither has been scientifically proven. Even so, Dark Matter was not known until very recently, neither did we understand water's magical properties or the fact that the human heart is supernatural (not subject to the laws of entropy). The most potent discoveries are those that prove the consciousness of our surroundings, such as ether, water, dust, plants and animals. With this information we can be inspired to discover the truth of our cellular structure as a means of understanding how to communicate with and reprogram the blessing that our bodies actually are. Perfect health is the most important possession. For without it, life becomes a drudgery of slavery to some form of painful imbalance.

As Gaia quivers in the wobble of Her divine precession, the collective human howl of urgency has struck the chord of panic. This is the very same panic that we struggle to forget. It is as old as instinct. Just how is our individual word contributing to this panoply of paradoxical double talk? When the inner message is different from the message we give outwardly, chronic imbalance establishes itself as normal and this is the real danger of the Battle of the Sexes. If our breath of life is not expressing our emotional truth, we have good reason to believe that we are riddled with guilt.

The difficulty with aligning our inner reality with our outer world comes from the lack of acceptance for the inner voice of disturbance that needs to spout off about the suppression that has been systematically imposed on the emotional body by a confused and frightened mind. The victim needs to speak to the perpetrator that has shamed the truth into hiding. Fortunately, for us, the human heart is capable of creating a sustainable and safe place for this transformation -- in this way we take responsibility for our condition and allow the un-evolved voices to speak without apology.

In the 20th century, the collective paradigm of humanity gave the technology of war to a global monster named Hitler. He was the sum total of our totalitarian God-concept that has led us to consider the "Fear of God" as a good thing. Fear of authority leads many loving souls into the darkness of deception. Fear of God comes from ancient ideas about karma that have more to do with power structures based on punishment, rather than education. I need only cite the fantastic imprisonment rates in the United States and the failing education system as a sad fact not to be denied further. As we have developed a new societal paradigm from a media that is exposing the true nature of the Human Condition, it is natural to wonder if the world is getting more violent when less people are dying from war today than any previous time in modern society.

Now, with "eyes everywhere" (the advent of cell phones with cameras), corruption is getting exposed as all there is to human society. I caution my fellows not to jump to conclusions about the world getting worse, instead, I would like to suggest that a great parting of the ways is in progress where honest people begin to separate from liars. If we are liars that override the Will of others, it is very reasonable to be frightened of reality because ultimately Providence only blesses balance. The guilt that embeds itself into the psyche of a personality that has chosen to lie to one's loved ones is a serious impediment to creating and maintaining electromagnetic balance that is capable of helping one maintain optimum physical, mental and emotional health that attracts like-beings. All who are in rejection of self to the point of chronic dishonesty will eventually cease to exist simply because the personality's own consciousness is in rejection of its own truth.

The most important choice a person can make is the choice to be honest to those around us and particularly with our selves. Just as water is able to mutate when subject to personality, likewise, daily decisions we make determine whether we create favorable conditions that enable one to maintain the Will to live. I started my life out as a liar and as a result of wanting to be a good mother, I decided to become the best person I could be. This helped me with my intimate relationships, but isolated me from many, many other opportunities. Many times I feel heartsick about the no-win paradigm the collective has formed to this point in our evolution. Ultimately, I believe in the power of love and know that my body responds very well to my burgeoning understanding of it, responds very well to my desire for life and my desire to contribute to the solution rather than deny the obvious imbalance. Feeling good about ones self is not a gimmick, it is a fine, unencumbered balance point that leads to breathing deep and making pro-life decisions that help us hum with the frequency of life.

OVERVIEW OF CHAPTER FIVE:

1. In the 1840's Michael Faraday discovered that oxygen is attracted to a magnet and is the GREAT PURIFIER that scrubs impurity from our body.

2. The human heart is not subject to entropy and does not fall apart or lose power over time.

3. The dominant paradigm causes the human heart to become subject to disease and entropy because of the electromagnetic repulsion that causes our resonant frequency to decline in a devolutionary manner.

4. Our WORD is heard by every cell in our body and when our inner word does not align with our outer word a dense form of nothingness (guilt) interrupts our electromagnetic matrix to end energetic reciprocity.

5. Secrets indicate the presence of shame and guilt and serve as a sort of Energetic Anti-matter that impairs energetic reciprocity and eventually causes a soul to lose the Will to live.

CHAPTER 6

YOU

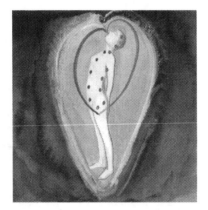

THE POWER OF PERSONALITY

What differentiates electromagnetism from Love? The involvement and prerogative of personality is what establishes the sentimental bonds of love. It is the cosmology of time and space to be responsive to consciousness and differentiated by personality and it is our ability to make moral decisions that gives humanity its spiritual prerogative. As we study the fundamental pattern of devolution, we will come to know our historic orientation to the ongoing Battle of the Sexes that has plagued us for approximately 13.5 billion years (this is the span of our collective birth and evolution of consciousness -- the approximate age of our Universe).

Presently, the acceleration of the earth changes is signaling the shift that will urge the masses to consider reality from a point of view that will bring them together to solve a common problem. It is now time to pull our selves together as individuals, and as a race. I do not wish to suggest that you must follow any particular criteria in order to create experiences that you desire because it only takes aligned desire. These issues will reveal themselves the longer one lives as the experiences that are necessary to help one clear his or her magnetic matrix come from the outer world. If, however, one would like to attend to clearing the magnetic blocks sooner then later, adopting the *Principle of Pangasm* can give adequate stimulation to bring the emotional body to the foreground for consciousness to accept and integrate within our heart, the center of our soul. The game offers a technique that clears blocks from our matrix in a dynamic and effective way compared to the alternative of waiting until our denial approaches us from the outer world to school us.

I do not like to be schooled about my own denial from outside of myself because I still have sensitivity to authority due to getting persecuted for having rebelled against authority in the past. This is why I am judicious about listening to the diverse points of view within my inner world as a means of creating consensus about what it is that I believe about myself and the world, and what it is that I want to experience. Quite often there is a war between these divergent points of view because of the indoctrination that estranges them into a confusing mess of self-doubt. However, the more I learn the truth about myself and the more I align my consciousness with my heart to establish emotional intelligence, the more I identify unique solutions. The denial that I come into contact with is always associated with blame or shame, both of which I take responsibility for. I am learning how to be my own authority and how to refrain from pushing my truth on others or allowing others to impose their truth on me. Sharing in an environment of honest intimacy looks and feels very different from the current competitive and defensive forms of communication that make us feel separate from one another.

Denial obscures the survival terror that forms as a result of projecting death for our future, crippling our ability to have True Free Will in regard to body function, sexual desire and lifestyle (among other things). If we are incapable of creating health, intimacy and belonging, we tend to also deny our seeming inability to create what we desire to the point of keeping the voice of our inner world a secret...especially since we are working overtime for acceptance from others after having lost precious self-acceptance. If this cycle goes on too long, the emotional body will do desperate things to relieve itself of this pressure, usually leading to attempts at more control on the part of the consciousness. This is a universal pattern that is related to by most of humanity as inevitable, convincing the masses to agree to stay silent, for the most part, about loneliness, perversion and injustice.

The pattern of self-rejection that covers up imbalance, instead of shining the light on the truth about imbalance, has developed our personality and our society. As we continue to live in a vacuum of self that distrusts self and the other, our body becomes twisted and the mind becomes a master manipulator...this is the end game of the Human Condition! The goal of Pangasm is to help us create agreement fields with others in order to open a safe Heart Space for denied negativity to have its day in court, so to speak. These sounds and emotions must express so that new information and emotions may come into this space to give form to our desired reality. Magnetic blocks can only be purged from our system through emotional (magnetic) movement/expression. This involves sound and body movement that enables the vibration that was originally denied to move through the matrix. The expression of denied magnetic blocks will enable one to attain the vibratory frequency necessary to flush the matrix and render it open and reciprocal.

Allowing the negative truth to speak has been an historic expression technique called "Exorcism". The fundamental difference between exorcism and the technique offered within the Principle of Pangasm is that exorcism puts the responsibility for the disturbance on an outside demonic presence while Pangasm recognizes the demonic expression of denied life as the responsibility of the personality expressing it. Denied negativity will silently stand by until it outgrows the conscious self in presence, making this disturbance seem as if it belongs to a different personality. Once this denied presence hits quantum mass (majority) it is able to kick our butt.

Through the mass hypnosis of the Battle of the Sexes, we have denied our truth to the point that we've lost the ability to feel and express the truth until such a time that the denied truth takes us over. In the absence of truth, we become so heartless through the repetition of self-rejection (suppressing our truth) that our personality faces extinction. Creating crisis through denying the truth is why the world is at war today. Self-awareness, matched by a willingness to become aligned, naturally leads us to release the denial by vibrating our truth and giving it acceptance this time...instead of more denial. As we express our denied emotions, the magnetic field becomes open and able to receive new information that can lead to evolving ever-increasing degrees of self-awareness and balance.

Many of you may remember an Arnold Schwarzenneger movie called *Terminator* with a villain that was a mutable gold liquid substance that could take on any form. Even after killing it in every imaginable way, this gold metallic man would reform once every last drop was re-capitulated, he then had the ability to take on any form he so desired...this is the same nature of Chi or the magnetic ether. It is truly a Genii in a bottle that is magnetized to your own special hearts code of personality. You do not have to take my word for this, I just ask you to contemplate the cartoon-like quality that modern civilization is reflecting through the billions of eyes we now have (cell-phones and the twitterpated collective consciousness) to witness the end-result of a 3rd dimensional paradigm that is currently the status quo Battle of the Sexes.

Fortunately, living in a State of Grace can only be achieved through absolute honesty. Those who are incapable of fundamental honesty will ultimately lose the Will to Live with the consequences of this damaging spiritual decision. As a result of the "sorting of the ways" preparation for Star-Gate, the illusions fostered by dishonesty will be replaced by reality, simply because Love is justice and mercy as expressed and experienced by personality. In a State of Grace, there is nothing that exists that is dishonest, we can take this at face value. We would not recognize our species if it were to achieve the 4th dimension of individual and collective consciousness. However, for now, in this relative 3rd dimensional state, it is helpful to open our heart to establish the agreement that it is even possible to achieve an aligned State of Grace in a body on earth.

Being sexual and having sexual intimacy is what gives life its intrigue and satisfying quality. To have health and love of life is wonderful, yet, sad if we have no one who we can share this with and no one to reciprocate our honesty and willingness. There is nothing I have ever experienced that compares to a simultaneous orgasm with one whom I love, and, having said that, it is important to stop planning our death if we want our orgasmic energy to co-create something other than cellular degeneration and a lack of intimacy. Changing the positive/positive or the negative/negative charge of Death Consciousness into a negative/positive reciprocal bond cannot be had through mental sophistries (ungrounded mental concepts) or we would be there already.

Holding magnetic emotional ether down and out from the heart stops the reciprocation of electric ether with its life partner the magnetic ether. Gold and silver sexing the 5 elements creates a dynamic presence of being that may seem alien to us after having been trapped in the anti-dynamic of devolution. Therefore, when emotional expression begins to move into the heart after having been suppressed, it requires a safe place to emote the shame and blame of imbalance without being made wrong for this truth.

During the latter half of the 20th century, emotional expression became a popular *"Gestalt"* method within the field of psychotherapy. Unfortunately, by only allowing extreme emotional expression without also adjusting the thought-forms that forced the imbalanced emotion to get stuck in the first place, will only damage the magnetic body further.

Undoing magnetic blocks that are held rigid by an unmoving magnetic field takes a willingness to utter the sounds of truth no matter whether they are negative or positive, loving or hateful. Emotional expression is the only way to unlock the magnetic matrix once the Battle of the Sexes gets installed. The counterpart of emotional movement is simply consciously releasing judgments that are founded in Death Consciousness. It is important to know that you are the only personality that may accomplish this vital counterpart to emotional release; judgment release is like untangling a web of self-delusion and it is helpful to understand that releasing these thought-forms opens the way for electromagnetic ether to flood the part of our matrix that was previously closed to this magical essence. It is essential to use our word in order to vibrate a change in the stuck thought-form that manipulated ideas in order to deny the voice of truth about chronic imbalance that is threatening our Will to live.

Our word comes from the air we breathe and our Heart Song is the wind beneath our wings capable of raising a personality out of devolutionary traps. In the past, the emotional counterpart of the mental polarity had been forced to conform to an unloving reality in the name of powerlessness and is generally unmoving because it has lost the Will to continue doing so within the context of the Battle of the Sexes.

The process of judgment release can be initiated in any number of ways. I usually back out of the trap by saying:

"I no longer believe that physical death is necessary" –

"I forgive myself for believing that my body must degenerate" –

"I no longer believe I was wrong when I chose to devolve" –

"I choose to believe that Free Will is my birthright", etc…

Our judgment patterns were derived from misunderstandings and serve to block our DNA from activating our true potential just as prison bars block desperate people from harming others or themselves. We cannot have super powers of divine proportion as long as we are operating with the Death Consciousness that denies life…nor should we.

The matrix of our particular pattern of D-Con is frozen in time and forces our space to begin closing in on us when our resonant frequency descends to such a low vibration that the parts of self begin to split apart. Devolution and the ensuing death of the body enables the suffering person to release the physical plane in the hopes of trying again in a different form with a new personality that has been largely shaped by the historic patterns of the past, yet again. This is evolution through the technique of death that most humans refer to as reincarnation. In other words, this process of evolution has been made possible through the use of devolutionary methods that establish a pattern of continual strife, similar to the age-old adage of: "Two steps forward and one step back."

The ability to establish balance and sustainability will eventually occur once the confines of devolution are cast away. Getting our emotional body to respond to our desire for life everlasting by re-magnetizing the upper and lower worlds into a viable positive/negative bond may feel futile, leading the person to feel foolish for daring to believe that magic is more than a fairytale in a children's book. Let me repeat myself here: desire IS the alchemy of magic.

The earthly map of separate communities that are competing for power demonstrates our devolving, collective god-concept that is looking for solutions through blame and shame; this paradoxical pattern is kept alive by the matrix of Death Consciousness, and almost the entire human race is presently enslaved within it, thereby, making earth the prison planet for the disease called war. We are the theater for the potential resolution of this collective misunderstanding about Providence and the human birthright of Personality.

Orgasm is the means by which we manufacture our experience in time and space as sexual personalities. Of course, ether travels our matrix at all times regardless of whether or not we are orgasmic, however, since orgasm delivers life force in an energetic flood capable of by-passing electromagnetic blocks, we generally feel some temporary relief from the rigid patterns of death after having an orgasm, even though the ether is not reciprocating on a normal basis.

By moving our life force through orgasm, we increase its substance exponentially, which is why serious imbalance for an individual begins to happen shortly after the first orgasm. This is the time when the matrix begins to feel the pressure of death and the ensuing Intimidating Form that persistently accompanies this paradigm.

Devolution has very real patterns that, if unchecked, always lead to our death. From an early age we begin to create rigid personality traits that are a REACTION to the dominant pattern of the expand/collapse cycle of devolution. Whether one is a rebel or a conformist depends on the willingness of the personality to accept injustice within the deepest levels of our psyche. These two limiting points of view appear as two equally limiting reactions. Suicidal or homicidal tendencies emerge when the Will to Live is threatened by intimidating form that is magnetically drawn to us as a regular feature of our individual and group paradigm. So regular that intimidating form has become the norm with very little trust or love to be found.

The reflection of Intimidating Form is presently escalating on a global level in that the mainstream of consciousness is hyper-aware of the prospect of global disaster, prompting discussion and movement toward legislation that addresses global issues; such as nuclear war, earth-changes and cosmic threats like asteroids, comets and solar weather. Since the group is devolving and immersed in Death Consciousness, the result of this "quickening" awareness of the collective is a quantum mass panic that is keyed to ancient and repetitive memories of group death, which is eventually the outcome of the group paradigm that firmly believes that death is inevitable. This linear paradigm creates a highly predictable pattern that robs individuals of the ability to perceive solutions that do not fall within the matrix of death. Under the influence of D-Con, the group develops sophistries about fate and "God's Will" that lead to a paradigm based upon human nihilism (hopelessness). Free Will has pro-life solutions once an individual aligns their heart with a desire for life that refuses to over-ride the Will of another.

Sexual shame is primordial to human society, faithfully handed down from one generation to another. In essence, we were born to confront this battle one way or another. Our species is looking at the issues surrounding sexual freedom and sexual fidelity from every perspective one can possibly hold in a world of time and space that is at war with itself. The resolution of this misunderstanding can more readily come about if we refuse to support the language of blame and shame, good or evil, right or wrong, etc. There is simply imbalance or balance and leaving the value judgments out of our communications will help those who are caught within the grips of imbalance to become willing to speak their truth about being in a compromising position. By coming out of the closet with our evolving point of view, no matter how un-evolved it may seem, we access our current truth with self-acceptance and openness. As stated previously, we must express the voice of blame and shame with the intent to release the judgments identified because of our emotional expression, not necessarily to direct blame at the other, but to identify the illusionary concepts that place responsibility for our reality outside of our self. Often, being harmed by another is a reflection of our own judgment field that makes us subject to this unfortunate pattern. Removing our selves from relationships and scenarios that are abusive is possible and desirable, therefore, moving back from those who would harm us or over-ride our Will is our responsibility. A judgment field that has been steeped in the ideas of good versus bad is a tricky dilemma, one that is best shared with other's that are also engaged in identifying D-Con judgments.

Creating a safe place for the marginalized voices of the inner realm to come out and argue, complain, moan and groan about what it has been like to be stuck in the Battle of the Sexes is the action of self-love. Acceptance of our truth is the only viable pathway to living within a State of Grace. Attempting to accept another that is calling guilt love is a confusing problem that will confuse us further as we adopt the guilt that is being offered as love. Having alignment with a sexual partner is powerful only so long as it does not produce more guilt or body shame. If guilt and body shame are denied, in order to have sex, this black magic creates any number of experiences designed to help us recognize that denial is threatening our existence. I hope you have enough love for your physical form to want to share it within a romantic embrace. If not, then finding a safe place to express the distress that naturally comes from being alone and facing the ugliness of aging to death is a good way to begin the emotional movement that is necessary to clear magnetic blocks within the Light Body.

This material is not addressing socio-paths who feel no remorse for over-riding other's, although I hold miracles up as the potential outcome for even the most damaged among us. Energetic magnetic blocks in our Light Body cannot be removed by simply choosing positive thinking or we would already be a world at peace with itself.

PRIMORDIAL GUILT (also known among Christians as *"Original Sin"*) cannot be addressed unless the thinking part is rescued from the endless downward spiral of devolution. Judgment release untangles the black magic of past patterns that are stuck in our cellular memory and presently troubling our heart. Emotional release either leads to judgment release or is a result of it, sometimes removing judgments can actually lead to emotional release. When I say a judgment release I pay attention to any body sensations that may occur, this is very good information about what part of our matrix is involved, kind of like mapping how our thought-forms get laid into our physical form. I have gone to great lengths not to impose my own relative judgment field into this information and want to remind you that the Principle of Pangasm is not about conforming to anyone else's ideas about what is real, instead, it is my intent that you develop ever greater degrees of understanding about the universal Laws of Nature as offering a virtually unlimited context within which to create a unique reality that pleases your heart.

This information is organized in such a way that you can make the intellectual connections to your individual matrix of self without so-called experts, gurus/priests or shrinks. The reason I categorize the archetypes of the 4 parts of personality as *Father, Mother, Son and*

Daughter is so that we may identify the relationships that we have on the inside with the relationships we carry on with others. The Spirit is consciousness and the Will is emotion, these two archetypes are the primary core of personality; if they are not in alignment then the secondary twin heart citadel of exchange, that is the Son and Daughter, never get to contribute anything that is productive to the creation. If North is not Sexing with South, then East and West go to war; die on the vine; wrestle for supremacy; etc. etc. etc. In this way we can see the patterns as archetypal and then we can word the judgment releases to better identify these universal patterns.

The issues of health and beauty are at the heart of Free Will and intimacy, (with our own body and within our relations to other people), is deeply affected by lack of health and beauty. If you find your body ugly or if your body does not respond to your attempts to have health and sexual interaction, it may be helpful for you to learn how to have sex with yourself as a way of creating health and beauty. However, this cannot happen if the personality is projecting death as their future transformative event.

Who would choose a body that does not please one's heart? I know that I would not choose a debilitated form or any reflection of ugliness, if I had a choice…and I do. However, after decades of devolution, I had received substantial damage that renders me ugly to my own eyes. Oh, it is wonderful when others tell me that I am beautiful and I could focus on my positive attributes as a means of trying to feel better about myself, but that approach to the reflection of ugliness is denial that is excluding the voice that is trying to point out the imbalance that is showing itself as ugliness. As you can see from this circular sentence, this is a loop much like a loop on a computer that stops all functions until the matrix is cleared of its gap. Usually, we turn it off and re-boot it - this is the same pattern as reincarnation…humankind evolving by means of devolution. We have been perpetually recreating ourselves through the technique of death, whereas, today, we have the means to discover the true responsive nature of the elements as a way of identifying our own superstitious thought-forms and evolving a more functional and humane paradigm. The Principle of Pangasm is a paradigm that glorifies the individual expression of Free Will while also potentially holding the larger group together in a State of Grace capable of sustainability.

The biological fact of *Pleomorphism* helps us understand that it is possible to heal our body in non-invasive, loving ways. When we understand that water is responsive to our self-concept, it becomes obvious that we are highly mutable. When we realize that the human heart is not subject to Entropy, we begin to grasp the power that a personality has to create life or death by way of Free Will. The key to establishing a balanced personality that enjoys an evolving perfection lies within making a whole-hearted agreement with this possibility.

The difference between "faith" and "trust" is similar to the difference between "fate" and "Free Will". Faith is a belief in an unproven reality while trust is belief based on fact and/or experience (it is experientially proven). Fate is perceived as a determining factor that comes from outside (i.e. divine intervention) while Free Will is the technique that one uses to determine ones own fate. Within the constraints of Free Will, the easy part is asking Creation for what it is that we want, whereas, the difficulty arises when we have inner conflict with what it is we may be asking for, or conflict with the possibility of even receiving our heart's desire.

Magnetic blocks in our Light Body can and will prevent one from aligning with their heart's desire simply because the block prevents the heart from being reciprocal between magnetic ether and electric ether in such a way that our heart is not conducting "L" energy. To the extent that blocks exist determines what access one has to their own heart and equally determines what types of experiences that individual is capable of magnetically drawing to self. Learning how to live within a society that lionizes death can "seem" more difficult than giving into death. Once I activated my Light Body through judgment release, and by feeling and expressing my unique truth, my Will began to operate in "seemingly magic" ways compared to the heartlessness I had become accustomed to! Now, after a decade of diligently taking responsibility for my denial, I have solid visceral evidence that this process saved my life and is healing my broken heart. No longer am I suicidal, although, I still do hear peripheral voices about "ending it all" from time to time, I simply take note and re-affirm my Will to live. Now, I relate to my body as a road map of the denial and the mercy that has brought me to the sublime solution of this revolutionary principle. In this manner I have substantially reversed the curse of D-Con and am rescuing my power from the pit of self-destructiveness.

Once alignment in our heart is our truth and our emotional body has the desire to move in the face of the intimidating form that says: "I am crazy to hope for mercy of this kind," then we can choose orgasm often with great appreciation that our body can deliver such a healing remedy free of charge! Upon orgasm many of us experience a rush of emotion… women often cry and men often pass out. This is a potent moment that could reconnect the emotional vortex to the heart through sound, movement, awareness and forgiveness. It is entirely helpful to vocalize the true emotional impact of our orgasm. If you are incapable of orgasm, then I suggest that you find a safe and private place to cry until you can move to touch your manifest body for some relief from the endless grief of a life without orgasm. For those who have never been able to achieve orgasm, it is recommended here that they seek professional help because this malady can come from a variety of emotional and physiological causes that defy generalization.

After a lifetime of battering our emotional body with shame and suppression, it is no wonder that it does not want to come out and express openly anymore because fear has polarized into terror, sadness into grief, and anger has become rage! Sometimes the emotional body is so beaten down by heartlessness that it is difficult to re-connect with, or take responsibility for, denied negativity like grief, terror or rage that essentially blocks access to our root. Whenever the emotional self attempts to clear itself of these extreme emotional polarizations, it has continually been met with shame and contempt on the part of the intellect, causing most all of us to re-double our efforts to repress our emotions. Control is an illusion that the mind uses as it tries to judge its experience before it actually happens, as a means of preventing error.

The attempt to control the future through more efficient means of manipulating the outer world will eventually cause disorientation because the mind is usurping its position when used in this way. The mind is not the organ that will assist in identifying the truth because that is not its function. The emotional body is designed to help us to feel the truth of our experience, whereas, the mind is the organ that performs the interpretive function about the experience after the heart expresses its emotional truth about said experience.

The *Principle of Pangasm* leads a soul into the invaluable contribution of a reciprocal Light Body aligned with the citadel of exchange between North, South, East and West in our human heart. However, the Battle of the Sexes disables the emotional body and puts the mind in the role of performing both functions of the emotions and intellect, leaving the heart with only one pole to derive its sustenance from. D-Con effectually starves the heart and collapses the channel of our electromagnetic Light Body. How's that for a vicious cycle?

What happens when we feel afraid and ashamed of our sexual expression? Sexual orgasm produces rapid magnetic pressure that rises up from our sexual center, so, if the matrix is blocked and the magnetic ether is unable to enter the heart, the magnetic ether arcs out of its matrix passing the block in order to integrate with the electric current that is moving down into the heart from the center of our brain. This creates a violent reality in the Light Body because the magnetic ether rushes in upon the heart, which had been stagnating without the motion of emotion up to the point of orgasm. Rather than integrate and align, the heart receives a tsunami of magnetic ether that has the force of violence, leading the conscious self to redouble its effort to control the emotional self through better discipline. Within the constructs of D-Con, moments of extreme emotion get interspersed with long moments of stagnation serving to cause one to lose the WILL TO MOVE the older one gets. We call these symptoms of an unmoving magnetic field laziness, depression and aging.

The method of violently arcing life force between the positive polarity and the negative polarity is the norm, which is why those polarized to the negative/negative eventually experience subtle or extreme forms of addiction, bi-polar disorder or schizophrenia. Actually, Bi-polar Disorder is the Human Condition in a nutshell, whereas, those who are polarized to positive/positive eventually become obsessed with being "right" and "in control" of those who are polarized to the negative polarity. This is an ongoing story of angels rescuing demons and demons destroying themselves, and, eventually, the angels as well. Schizophrenia is the result of arcing between North and South as a means of trying to fill the vortices of East and West with electromagnetic ether. These psychological maladies are studied deeply, yet at this time, the only clinical solution is to drug the disturbed, smack dab in the middle of a war on drugs. Talk about confusing!

Flipping from one pole of our being to the other is what heartlessness creates...a violent energetic conundrum that renders the personality unsustainable as it only has access to either the upper or lower parts of their Light Body. This ping-pong of exchange will exhaust the Will to Live because of the persistent violence that breaks apart the personality when it is under this type of duress for any length of time.

Under the influence of D-Con, every orgasm requires a recovery time to revitalize the Light Body with ether. Since D-Con is linear, the loop of infinity (that is the citadel of the heart's exchange matrix) breaks apart and becomes a linear channel that bleeds ether out the crown. The older one gets, the more difficult it becomes to raise the sexual vibration for more of the same violence that persistently produces disappointment and disillusionment that we call cynical or heartless.

When one is chronically out of balance, emotional honesty is a tricky paradox to navigate in a culture that lionizes death as the great reward for living while sanctioning dishonesty as a rational survival technique. The pattern of allowing our intellect to dictate what we should be feeling is the hallmark of D-Con and after years of rejecting our truth in this manner, it is hard to identify what it is we actually feel anymore. Most of our emotional movement is in a reactionary state to the death urge, therefore, we have never really known what a balanced heart can feel like or produce.

The shame affecting the sexuality of humanity comes from the collective misunderstanding about sexual ether, its properties, how it moves and how to utilize this ether without creating imbalance. Our rigid rules, traditions and laws regarding sexuality are a reflection of this misunderstanding. We have judged ourselves harshly and, as a result, many people begin their sexual relationships with secrets, body-shame and a deep-abiding fear of being found out, a deep abiding fear of being abandoned or held hostage. On top of this, we were never told that our orgasmic ether was not circulating in a proper way. There is so very much we have not been told about orgasm that the word itself is used in hushed tones.

Please allow me to recap this critical issue: when orgasmic ether begins to move up to the heart, the portals of our matrix must be open to complete the exchange of electric ether with magnetic ether. In the presence of guilt, the portal of electromagnetic exchange between the root and crown (the heart) closes its access gate with an invisible mass that I call "*The Rock of the Tomb*." Emotional ether hits this block like a wave smashing against a solid barrier. This lack of reciprocity is happening on subtle levels at all times, however when orgasm is occurring this same ether hits the block with exponential force. This anti-dynamic magnetically draws intimidating form that is designed to help the person in denial recognize their self-rejection, guilt and debilitated position. This is the nature of denial. It does not just slap us up side the head in order to make us pay for our sins. Most people believe this is how karma works. However, the negative experience is not a punishment because the strife is simply a message about imbalance.

If we could identify imbalance, in order to help us recognize our misunderstandings about the Laws of Nature and the nature of personality, we could then evolve into a more centered place of existence making it possible to create pleasure instead of pain. Evolution does not require pain, suffering or sacrifice in order to progress. The misunderstandings that have created persistent patterns of pain and suffering have led to the collective idea that it is virtuous to sacrifice ourselves as a means of building character. We can get what we want without suffering, while at the same time develop our character, because life was meant to be pleasant not some continuous war that crushes the Will to Live out of us for goodness sake!

The sound that comes forth from our breath of life is our Time/ Space signature and has tremendous physical implications. If you are in physical pain while reading these words, you can have instant relief by using your breath to moan. That's right… if you are in pain, moan into the pain as you stretch your body. This is a visceral solution that is available to you anytime without the need for money, doctors, transportation or medicine. The vibratory sound from moaning will remove blocks from the body such as lactic acid and energetic blocks from the Light body, such as guilt. If your physical pain motivates you to moan for relief, then you have learned the best of instant remedies that will ALWAYS BE AVAILABLE - FOR FREE - as long as you can breathe and make sound! Note: moaning is not necessarily a means of resolving the cause of pain it simply postpones pain until the cause of the pain is identified. Removing the belief that "the body must deteriorate" is a good place to begin healing from D-Con. Once a person establishes a healthy Will to live, then they can embark on the path of recovering their physical form from a lifestyle that was founded on heartlessness toward our body. Our sound will clear the blocks from our matrix once we genuinely choose life with our incarnate body. The seeming non-response that our body has given in the past, when we wanted it to perform some function, isn't because the body is unresponsive to our desire, instead, the non-responsiveness of our mortal body is caused by the congested Light Body that was disrupted through our chronic emotional suppression while under the influence of the Battle of the Sexes.

The magnetic field is only capable of the movement necessary to pull itself back together when there is a Will to live that is strong enough to eclipse the previous plan for death.

The plan for death has put into place a debilitated emotional response that is under the influence of hopelessness presently called acceptance. Forcing oneself to accept chronic imbalance that is creating a reflection of injustice, violence, debilitation and death is like selling one's Soul. Our Soul is quite literally the magnetic aspect of our personality that we use to attract our experience, human magnetism/charisma. Our magnetic matrix has a code that is responsive to our unique heart. It is possible to have our magnetic ether entangled with that of others through the unholy agreements of D-Con as these unholy agreements are the norm and have given rise to forms of energetic theft instead of reciprocal sharing.

Suppressed emotional response is holding consciousness in a separate state from the heart. We have identified this separation by realizing that there is the conscious mind and the sub-conscious mind. These are two seemingly non-communing entities in the same body that are fighting for dominance. The sub-conscious self represents the denied consciousness that was forced to stay silent. When denial becomes larger than the consciousness, denial owns the personality. It is around this time that the grim reaper becomes willing to claim that which we are in denial of.

Denied survival-terror can and will create intimidating form as a way of pressuring us to identify the original cause of the suppressed expression of our truth. This is the state that desire is in today and it has been demonized and pushed into hell. Blame, shame and loneliness are the only result of keeping our truth secret. Loss of vibration is the result of rejecting our emotional truth behind the belief that says: "There is nothing that can be done to change the relentless patterns of loss and death." This is why depression in Western civilization is currently pandemic causing mothers to kill their own children, fathers to murder the mothers of their children, workplace and church massacres, children murdering their parents and classmates, and prisons that are full of the impoverished.

Intimidating form is the backlash of suppressed emotional movement coming back to us from the outer world after having been rejected within the inner world. If this pattern of transference from the inner world to the outer world were in a state of balance, it would bring our heart's desire to us in the form of experiences that we want to have. When we are in denial of our desire, self-rejection boomerangs out from and back to, in order to inform us of our fundamental misunderstanding about the innate power of personality which we are actively denying. This is the circular paradox of the 3rd dimension while under the influence of D-Con.

Being a spiritual personality in a physical body has built-in support within the Laws of Nature that had not been previously known. We had, as a species turned to superstitious ideas to help us make sense out of a brutal reality that does not seem to support our free Will. It is reasonable to fall into the trap of blame and shame for being subject to the type of brutality that has always punctuated our societal groupings and families. However, now that science is uncovering the innate lovingness of Providence, as grounded in the scientific truth about the elements that support our existence, we can shed superstitious blame and shame to enter into a new reality that many are today calling the New Age.

OVERVIEW OF CHAPTER SIX:

1. It is our ability to make moral decisions that gives personality its spiritual prerogative.

2. Through the mass hypnosis of the Battle of the Sexes, we have denied our truth to the point that we've lost the ability to feel and express the truth until such a time that the denied truth takes us over.

3. After a lifetime of battering our emotional body with shame and suppression, it is no wonder that it does not want to come out and express openly anymore because fear has polarized into terror, sadness into grief, and anger had become rage.

4. When orgasmic ether begins to move up to our heart, the portals of our Light Body matrix must be open to the flood of energy that is orgasm, in order to complete the exchange of electromagnetic ether.

5. Intimidating form is the backlash of suppressed emotional movement coming back to us from the outer world after having been rejected within the inner realm.

CHAPTER 7

The Game of panGasm

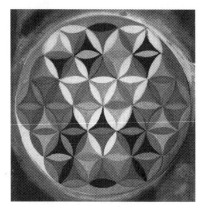

PLAY

The pressure that comes from intimidating form increases with time as it threatens our loved ones and our own life. Scientific information about the physical plane combined with metaphysical information about the spiritual plane can help us piece together this macrocosmic matrix of the broken heart as a way of identifying our own individual orientation to this pattern. Heartlessness has reached such a quantum mass for humanity that we are threatening worldwide annihilation by means of the very same technology that is simultaneously knocking upon our door to educate our consciousness to help bring about resolution.

The *"War on Terror"* is as insane as the *"War on Drugs"* that is attempting to prevent our use of numbing agents we ingest to help us deny our survival terror. Why is the United States addicted to self-destructive drugs and alcohol? To help us cope with denied or not so denied terror. This paradoxical insanity will confuse anyone into compromising their own values in the face of hopelessness that says there is no solution other than acceptance and compromise… nothing like dancing with the devil!

The value structure that we have adopted as a result of the Battle of the Sexes is really a list of various attempts to cope with the no-win dogma of planning ones death. As a result, our personality gets cut off from the genuine evolutionary development that would have given us the ability to create a satisfying life and the acceptance from others that we crave. If we make honesty the first habit and non-violence the first rule, then the way opens up for our truth to come out of the closet and express its particular form of distress. This is why the language of shamelessness that the principle before you provides is a great beginning as it leads us to create agreements with others that sanction the creation of a safe place for our denied negativity to express itself. I call this agreement HEART SPACE. This agreement between two or more people creates a tangible reality that feels safe to the soul, which was forcing itself into non-existence through continual self-rejection and silence about the chronic imbalance that stems from D-Con.

Heart Space is a viable container for the clearing of suppressed and depressed magnetic ether to come forward and deliver the message about imbalance. The Heart Space created by this type of agreement sets the stage for True Free Will to evolve through self-acceptance and openness. Sharing our truth with others who are also taking responsibility for imbalance will help us feel safety. However, this feeling of safety and trust has been absent while under the influence of the Battle of the Sexes. This explains why cynicism has formed our relations. In fact, once we begin to express the unmoving denied magnetic charge as un-evolved emotional movement, we will have tangible evidence of how powerful this force is, especially if we replace the thought-forms of death with the thought-forms of self-determination (True Free Will).

In my own experience, adopting this paradigm gave me renewed health while reversing the effects of aging. No kidding! Just as I was beginning to look haggard from heartlessness, I began to move the denied emotional congestion and watched my body transform. Today, I am still dealing with decades of denial that are reflected by physical distress and I relate to this as a process of accessing my root, one day at a time. I still have knee-jerk moments of distrusting my body and believing it will die, no matter how much I release judgments and emotions, but, I choose to understand that intimidating form is tantamount in this world and I am in the vanguard of this movement, meaning the loneliness and separation I feel is also part of my healing process, part of the layers of intimidating form I had laid into this form since childhood. Since I have had tangible good results from adopting this paradigm, I have chosen to have a persevering faith in love. It is this faith in love that pleases my heart and fuels my dreams.

My orientation to the upper and lower worlds is Heart centered today as a result of taking responsibility for the guilt that kept me oriented to the dark pole of the feminine force… constantly blaming Yang. As a representative of the divine feminine polarity of the darkness, I now want to shed light on how this rebellion has formed our governments and religions. I bring this up now to give you a sense of what created religious thought on earth and why women are demonized and forced into myriad forms of prostitution as a means of survival. Essentially, women around the world could stop the wars that are raging if they understood their power and resolved the split in their inner world...first and foremost!

The most important sexual issue to come from the battle between the Yin and Yang is what happens to a woman when she has sex with a man who is in denial of his guilt, fear, rage and hopelessness. When a woman takes a man into her body to consummate sexual exchange, she takes in all of his denied, and not-so-denied self-rejection. Then, she energetically produces his denied self-concept into physical form. In effect, when we mix our personalities in the act of sexual intercourse, the forms of self-rejection we are holding in a state of denial will translate into the outer world to inform us of such. This pattern of denial is how we collectively created hell on earth through orgasm in the presence of guilt and denied negativity.

We have joined in agreement to gather on this planet and renegotiate our paradigm much like the cells in our body collaborate to vibrate health or morbidity. You are reading these words in this moment because you have become ready to mutate your vibratory field into a position that matches the new frequency that the earth is resonating… if you haven't already. This information is already vibrating around the world in different forms and styles to assist all those who love life to separate out from those who project death into their physical form; to separate from the truly self-destructive persons that could influence our Will to live in a detrimental way. Those of us who are developing the ability to separate out from death may do this without having to act outwardly in opposition to anyone or anything. This process has been turbulent up until now because of the intimidating form that our collective Death Consciousness has formed over the millennia, as a result of our collective denial of life. Truly, the only outward action we need to take, in order to heal this paradox, is the art of caring for our physical form and providing for its basic needs. Of course money is involved in this endeavor and our personal relationship with money will help us to identify our position to the rebellion against authority: The Battle of the Sexes. When we begin to recognize our own orientation to this linear paradigm, we will then have information about our belief-structure in such a way that we can undo the unholy thought-forms that keep us trapped in the linear realm of self-rejection.

There really is no conspiracy to speak of that is working against our freedom, it is the natural result of our paradigm. We have the ability as individuals and as a collective family to stand present while the denial of life leaves this realm, once we agree to be honest with one another. In the past, those of us who are "Love Incarnate" developed a misunderstanding about the difference between life and death. This misunderstanding prompted love to hold on to death in the name of love and life, whereas each individual has developed since this agreement-field was formed, according to their own unique brand of D-Con judgments that I call "*Original Cause*." The goal of this game is to offer you the tools necessary to discover your own "original cause" and design your unique belief structures to be in synchrony with the Laws of Nature as well as your own personal desires. If your personal desire does not match with the group you currently interact with then you may have a reflection about your "original cause" as a way of helping you to identify whether you rebel against authority or conform to it. In the past, dictates came down from the consciousness instead of up from the root, our Will; this is backwards, as it is the function of the human Will to select the experience. This is why we live in an apparently evil condition with little freedom of choice. What this means to you will be yours to determine.

This game has very few rules and a very specific goal which is to help the participants clear the magnetic blocks gained from denying our emotional negativity, such as: survival terror, denied righteous indignation, denied shame, denied rage, denied hopelessness, etc., thereby, restoring the reciprocity between the crown and root (Heaven and Earth). By clearing these energetic pathways of the human Light Body, we can open space for life to begin flowing from North to South and East to West in the spiral dance that enables a sexual body to make love and co-create experience, as well as, procreate more people in our likeness...if we so desire.

THE most important rule is that the players solemnly agree not to engage their genitals during this game. If the desire to have sex is agreed upon by both parties as a result of coming together to play, it is still understood that touching each other's genitals will not happen during this particular meeting. In other words, agree to meet another time for sexual engagement after you have slept in separate locations. When we come together for this game we will definitely bring up some highly volatile essence, therefore, it is necessary to create a solid agreement field that sex (including oral sex) will NOT occur as a result of playing Pangasm. We do not wish to trick the Desire Body/Emotional Self to come out for something it wants only to deny it again, because this is potentially harmful for this part of us since denial of authentic emotional response is all it has ever known. Sex is not bad, dirty or shameful, however, if there is no HEART SPACE between partners about what sexual interaction means for this relationship, then it is simply mutual masturbation that does not include our whole self. Casual sex does not heal the heart! Instead, it reinforces self-doubt because intimacy rarely occurs as a result of this type of un-grounded sexual desperation. Pangasm is not for you if you do not wish to engage your whole heart within your sexual interactions!

Sexual orgasm in the presence of guilt is deadly, PERIOD!

This is a game that can have lasting effects on our Soul. It can be fun, and it is also helpful to be serious about the commitment that we make to the few rules of Pangasm if we are actually to benefit from this therapeutic technique.

Many people still waste money hiring a psychiatrist and then lie to that person because self-acceptance has become non-existent for them. Anyone can continue the devolutionary game of trashing their heart, and one can find a lot of company that will support shredding our heart because humanity collectively believes that life is about loss and death. However, the undercurrent of those that live this way is one of guilt that is under tremendous pressure from systematically denying their truth, denying their authentic expression and from orgasm in the presence of guilt.

True Free Will leads to sexual freedom between consenting adults, however, if denied shame is gone past in order to have sexual freedom, the backlash can lead to forms of hopeless desperation that I do not wish upon anyone.

We do not need to maintain the values of others in order to heal our heart, but we do need to know what our own values are so that we may be true to ourselves. Most all of us have learned values from those who are under a lot of pressure from guilt and lack of self-acceptance. Those who taught us the paradigm of D-Con are not *wrong* for having been taught this as children themselves, and therefore passing this along, but now that we understand that the Laws of Nature truly support Free Will, it is up to us to break the hold of D-Con by choosing to align our whole self with life.

Sexual attractiveness is not in the eyes of the beholder, since we are the only person in creation that matters when it comes to looking into the mirror and loving our form enough to expose it. Even if we are able to attract others who find our form attractive when we do not also find our own form attractive, we are only denying our truth by looking outside of our self for acceptance from the other as a means of going past our own body-shame. Having a deep desire to love our physical form will help us to locate and emote the truth of what it feels like to be seemingly powerless when it comes to health and beauty. "Mirror" therapy is an affective technique to find denied body-shame. As you view your naked form, inspect your expression, look into your eyes and see what feelings are there. Allow the voice of shame to begin expressing everything you dislike about your form. As you do this, listen for the rigid judgments about your form and your perceived inability to influence it, and then, release these judgments in whatever manner you are capable.

The emotional body is the key to liberating our Heart from the confines of time and space. Both positive and negative emotions are necessary to maintain the full spectrum of emotional vibration that enables us to balance our physical self with the 4 parts of personality into an aligned vehicle that is self-sustaining. Rather than trying to hypnotize our emotional-body with ungrounded positive thoughts that deny the negative points of view, it is good to express the negativity with a healthy dose of understanding for the part of self that had to remain silent in the name of presenting false balance when, in fact, imbalance was the truth. Those who go past the subconscious guilt regarding chronic imbalance in order to engage in casual sex are opening to a form of "Russian Roulette" (a gambling form of suicide) that will leave the Soul bankrupt with shame.

Removing our self from the vicious cycle of chronic self-rejection will feel dangerous, futile, frightening, frustrating, etc., and all of these feelings, and more, are the key to clearing our energetic matrix of death, so open to these lifesaving vibrations with a healthy dose of respect for the feminine polarity of negativity. I must repeat that the polarity of negativity is not absent of love -- it has simply been demonized by a long-standing misunderstanding. Emoting denied negativity will bring up all the shame and blame that had been pressuring us to present a false persona, this is not an endless process, but at times may feel like it is; this is why it is good to find others that understand this process of magnetic clearing and can support us when we reach the root of the disturbance; therefore, the game is designed to help us find these others that can support our heart in times of need.

Expressing the un-evolved voice of the denied emotional disturbance may sound ridiculous, foolish, childish, hateful, jealous, etc., however, once the emotional self begins to move after having been stuck, we will come face to face with our denied truth because this is where we left it. In order to reintegrate this lost emotional expression, we must give it a safe place to GET REAL. Once we get the magnetic ether moving (you will know when this is occurring because you will feel the vibration of emotion moving through your body), we need to let our sound erupt as a way of opening the channel from top to bottom...essentially vibrating our space open for the light (crown) to come into the body (root) and raise the resonant frequency to match that of earth...this is *Heartsong*. As this occurs, you will have a flood of ideas and images coming into your consciousness. So, listen closely because this is where we find the D-Con thought-forms that hold us trapped in the 3rd dimension of devolution.

The Pangasm technique for using sound is a language of the heart that I call *VAGARIAN*. This universal language bypasses the interpretive function of the mind because it is the language of the emotional body. Anyone can learn this language instantaneously because there is no wrong way or right way to express Vagarian. You may know this language as Gibberish or as *"speaking in Tongues,"* etc. This is a usage of sound in a non-lingual manner that expresses emotions without words; it can be sung, screamed, grunted, whispered or moaned and comes from your breath of life in a nonsensical manner. Of course, if you desire, you can use words because identifying our emotions with words is sometimes helpful as well. Whether through words or Vagarian sounds, it is important to make sound when the moment of ignition occurs because the heartsong will, through re-creating the vibration of the previously denied expressions, recalibrate our electromagnetic matrix to become reciprocal.

One of the primary requirements for the success of this dating game is within the moment of *IGNITION*. In order to reach ignition, the two participants must share a mutual sexual attraction for one another. This game does not work if sexual attraction is not present on the part of both participants. Besides, it is cruel to the other and abusive to the self to force self to pretend attraction for a person who is attracted to us. The *Principle of Pangasm* is not meant to help us perpetuate heartlessness, but, on the contrary, it is meant to untangle the matrix of denial that naturally comes from the Battle of the Sexes. Ignition is something that cannot be faked because it is the honest response to mutual sexual arousal. Ignition happens when one or both participants feel such extreme pressure to have sexual intercourse that they are willing to break the rules of this game.

Ignition creates a moment when, one or both players have access to their crown and root simultaneously. This is a potentially therapeutic opportunity to activate the heart and establish reciprocity between the crown and root of our previously separate Light Body. Within this game, our body is the tool and mutual sexual desire is the currency that opens the crown and the root (Heaven and Earth) for our hearts to align with life.

THE GAME

THE RULES:

First, there is the invitation. You can customize this with flowers, poetry, pastry or my favorite…chocolate! This is an opportunity to express your unique personality. This book can serve to be the invitation that you give to your chosen date. It is important for your partner to understand the principle so the game can serve as a therapeutic healing modality; this is the reason the book is written in the order provided; by understanding the principle the participants can apply this to the game to make it a therapeutic event.

The fear that arises from such a brave move as to offer this principle to another person as a viable pathway to intimacy is, in itself, a therapeutic trigger. For it is within this moment of fear and self-doubt that we have a rare opportunity to find many of the Original Cause thought-forms that block our pathway to experiencing the kind of intimacy that we crave.

Second, secure a location that is private and has a bed or a clean floor with a blanket over it. If you are out doors, make sure you have shade and shelter from the elements and bugs. Ambiance is nice, such as a fire, soft lighting, music, etc. Tea or wine is fine…whatever you like. This is a creative moment that will set you apart from the rest of the people in the world. Please know that Pangasm does not ever recommend any form of synthetic drugs (pharmaceuticals, ecstasy, crack, cocaine, L.S.D. or anything made in a lab by someone you never actually met). These types of drugs are serious self-destructive aids. Besides, drugs will mask our truth and since the goal of the game is to understand how our electromagnetic ether moves and feels, it is important to feel our truth instead of the drugs we may choose to ingest. Besides, **this game can and does help the body to make the best drugs known to mankind**. Our Limbic System produces endocrines that supply THE best drugstore in the world. The glands in our body can, and will, produce the effects of an expensive street drug known as ecstasy. This game provides an empowering opportunity to learn how to feel good without harming our physical body or compromising our sexual values. This method of creating our own ecstasy through stimulating our body's chemistry is free, legal, safe and fun…it is, quite simply, our glorious birthright.

Third, wear comfortable clothing and make sure you have unhindered movement in these clothes because some of us like to play Pangasm like Olympic wrestlers for goodness sake! Just make sure that you cover the genitalia with something that won't slip open --it is agreed that the genitalia may not play. This is the most important rule of the game and establishes a remorse-free zone where sexual energy may be conjured up to entertain, heal and inform us of what type of power is available to us at all times.

Fourth, give yourself a lot of time with no interruptions. Turn off the cell phones, put out the pets, etc. Have the children in a separate location and make sure you can make lots of noise without worrying about what the neighbors might think. It is important that you and your partner have no appointments between the meeting and a full night's sleep afterwards.

How to begin…

Converse about the ground rules of Pangasm and the contents of this book and share any fears or insecurities, as well as any desire that is felt toward one another -- sharing about what it is that attracts you to each other. Map these emotions and hook up to them because they are the guard at the door that will initiate your access to emotional ether! Anticipation, fear, shyness, insecurities and especially mention what it was like leading up to this moment…from the time of invite. This reflection offers insights into each other's inner world and opens the space for intimate interplay.

Blindfolds, although optional, are spectacular fun because they make us approach experience from an orientation we are unaccustomed to and serve to help us feel on deeper levels. Also, body shame can relax if ugliness is not seen. The fact that we take the genitals out of play helps to make the whole body an erogenous zone and disengaging sight will help tactile touch to take on a whole new realm of awareness.

My favorite position to initiate Pangasm is to sink into my partner's arms with my head on his shoulder, breathing in each other's presence and coming into awareness of what it feels like to be with this individual, versus, how it feels to be alone. In your day-to-day normal reality, I recommend spending ample time alone lying on your back, indulging in what it feels like to be in your body. Register every little sensation and get accustomed to your vibratory field, your breath and the beating of your heart. This way, when you do lay with someone, you can easily tell the difference in vibration and whether this change is pleasant or uncomfortable.

At no time is violence an acceptable form of expression. As well, rapists belong in jail. Have a reasonable idea about whom you are with. Let others know you are there with this person in an intimate setting and know the person's last name, telephone number, etc.

Prior to healing our Hearts, we can oftentimes attract extreme, out-of-balance situations, which are essentially designed to inform us of our denials and can serve to make any situation a potential hazard… such as driving a car.

I am not telling you this to frighten you, but do remember that you have been planning your death for some time. So, open to the messages that fear wants you to receive and then find a safe place to verbally express your fear -- for this too is a potent expression to allow into the initial moments of play. You will learn much about your personal patterns that allow for valuable insight to your Original Cause. It is the voice of disturbance in our inner world that holds the clues to our un-evolved self-concept. Once we begin to listen for these insights, we can make a point of releasing these judgments as if they were actual bricks in an invisible prison that keep us separate from one another.

Now that it is understood that the two of you are meeting for a righteous make-out session and the agreement is solidly formed that no sexual intercourse or oral sex will occur during this session, it is time to allow nature to take its course. Once the sexual ether begins to move as a result of touch and desire, you will begin to notice a drug-like state of being that feels lighter and less limiting and laughter often occurs. Take your time and revel in every little nuance of sensation because sexual affection accentuates all of our senses, especially our extrasensory sixth-sense that is clairvoyance.

It is fine to converse, cajole, tease, rant, growl, tickle, caress, kiss and wrestle. There are definite stages to the acceleration of sexual ether and I do not recommend speeding past any of the stages. Eventually, the interaction will create an ignition point. Ignition is the moment when one or both people feel as though they absolutely need to take this game to the next level...sexual penetration and orgasm. Instead of following our need to have sex, it is at this juncture of ignition where the therapeutic aspect of the game can occur.

It is so very much fun to save the ignition experience for later, rather than sooner. You can do this by agreeing to back away from the pressure to 'go for it' by deep breathing and the use of Vagarian and then, of course, we always laugh at the point Vagarian establishes the game. Then, we start to wind the sexual desire back up toward another ignition. Moving slowly is a great way to feel every little sensation of exchange. The blessing is that we arranged our time in such a way that there is no outside pressure forcing us to move in any other way than we desire. Of course, we are all different and sometimes fast and furious is what the chemistry is about. I do not wish to create many limitations, except for the obvious limits against engaging in oral sex, groping genitalia or intercourse.

As far as violence and name-calling goes, these are areas some people may be open to experiencing, especially if they were mistreated in these ways in the past. Those who are interested in this type of therapy, and before the game begins, can make agreements with one another that violence should be expressed as name-calling, cursing, etc., because, using violence in this game as a healing modality is too dangerous. I recommend professional therapy for this level of disturbance. Within this form of sexual interlude is a dance as varied as the potential players and should always honor the participants as we acknowledge the innocence of the mutual desire we hold for one another.

From the moment of invitation to the actual moment of embrace is a part of the dance that is Pangasm. Even getting rejected by a person that you invite is part of the healing process designed to align the human Light Body with life by routing out the thought-forms of self-rejection. Feeling the truth of our existence is the only way to begin the magnetic clearing that I am suggesting. Rejection from the outer world is always a sign of self-rejection coming back at us from our inner world. So, take responsibility by feeling the depth of rejection and identifying the thought-forms that have decided you are not worthy of reciprocal attraction...for whatever reason.

The goal of ignition is also an individual choice. If, at any moment, a part of us becomes so uncomfortable we cannot move forward, then make sounds and disengage from one another until one or both parties are no longer overwhelmed or choose to end the meeting with Heart-space that knows no urgency to stuff any preconceived events into one meeting...or at least, not this one. If your game ends prematurely before ignition, please, in this particular situation, allow disappointment to register emotionally after you have parted ways. For many of us, genuine emotional expression is disturbing, especially if it is directed at us – and the feelings of overwhelm should be respected and not pressured further.

In this game, we take responsibility for our own disturbance by helping to remind each other that we are not responsible for anything other than our own feelings. Normally, when we are disturbed, blame and shame show up to help us displace the negative emotions that are pressuring our heart for expression, since most all of us have been taught that negative emotions are wrong to indulge in. We have been un-accepting of the negative pole of expression for so long that, to some, we appear ugly during the expression of this demonstration of extreme emotion. Pay attention because this is a dynamic opportunity for self-awareness that could help reverse the paradoxical trap of denial that comes from feeling wrong about feeling negative emotions, such as blame and shame.

It is a natural response to want to blame and shame others, directly or indirectly, if we meet with disappointment because D-Con has delivered it so regularly that we feel as though we are at a breaking point when disappointment comes back around in its seemingly endless cycle. And, it is important not to make others responsible for the way we feel (unless, they have harmed us by over-riding our free Will) because the Heart Space that was created by coming together to play this game is in the spirit of blamelessness... no matter how disturbing the event may become. Awareness of our core sexual truth, even if we do not like what we become aware of, is a vital component of aligning the four parts of personality. Learning why we originally denied these parts of our self is how we identify D-Con thought-forms, then we may consciously release them with our word – doing this together can be fascinating and comforting. Rituals that release the black magic of Death Consciousness judgments are powerful actions capable of placing the parts of self on the same page. Over all, I like to keep things simple. Our word is sound and color in motion so let the sound move during the game.

If all systems are "full speed ahead" and sexual ether is beginning to flood the room, notice how the lighting, colors and atmosphere of the space change. Discuss sensory observations with one another throughout the game as a way of getting to know how electromagnetic ether under the influence of extreme sexual desire can affect us when it is free from shame.

Ignition happens when one or both parties feels as though they must have sexual intercourse or else! The moment of ignition is generally the moment when, under normal circumstances, most of us break our sexual rules... if we have any. This is one of the most dynamic opportunities of sexual healing available and is a highly volatile one too.

It is in the moment of ignition that the North, South, East and West (our entire being) simultaneously open to our command. "OPEN-SAYS-ME!"

When the channel is open from our root to our crown, the conscious mind and the sub-conscious mind become as one. This is an amazing event! No matter who you are, what gender you are, how young or old you are, how pretty or ugly you may be, rich or poor, sick or healthy, analytical or emotional, positive or negative...it does not matter. If you reach ignition, you have moved Heaven and Earth and they are all eyes, ears and open hands awaiting your command. Time to express the truth, the whole truth and nothing but the truth! The goal is to bring the emotional expression out of hiding to express itself in an environment of acceptance for it, in an environment of shamelessness.

If this moment was prepared for and agreed upon initially when the rules of the game were discussed, the Heart Space of agreement can lead the players through a portal of self-awareness that is capable of moving blocks from our Light Body matrix. Simple sound and body movement can serve to express any ecstatic joy, pain, frustration, gratitude, anger, sadness, playfulness, JOY, fear, happiness, grief, rage, JOY, terror, love, lust, depression, JOY, and don't forget the absolute JOY of feeling passionate LIFE FORCE moving through our body.

In the moment of ignition, sexual pressure dwells. This is the opportunity to move old emotional charges so that we may align in the present moment of the unified 9th dimension. This dimension is achieved when the 4 parts of personality (inner world) align with the 5 elements (outer world) of our earthly existence. Achieving an aligned 9th dimension as personality is a *State of Grace* (known as the *Wu Wei* in Buddhist tradition) and this moment of ignition is the pinnacle of opportunity to access our entire being for alignment, especially the sub-conscious and unconscious selves that we generally have no conscious access to except in a dream state, hypnosis or moments of crisis. This event is the simultaneous opening of the upper world of conscious intelligence to the lower world of emotional vibration. Unfortunately, the current human condition had established emotional imbalance, so be prepared to open PANDORA'S BOX and let the contents spill out with a healthy dose of acceptance.

We never really know what will come up for us emotionally when ignition occurs for one or both participants. Sometimes it is uncontrollable laughter while at other times it could be blaming rage, extreme sadness, frustration or shame. We don't really know, nor should we try to limit our experience by projecting a planned response. There needs to be agreement between the parties about creating Heart-Space for whatever comes up in this moment (except for physical violence).

Within the context of Pangasm each person is considered an equal. We share ourselves instead of minister to one or the other (ministry connotes a 'better-than -- less-than' imbalance, instead of one human sharing love and truth with another for free). We really do not need someone to fix or rescue us as much as we need genuine intimacy where one person shares in the spirit of honesty as much as the other. If you are making an admission of some sort where you are revealing a sensitive issue, do you want reciprocation, as in the other revealing his/her self in like style? Reciprocation of intimacy in a setting of honesty and acceptance creates understanding and compassion. Or do you want someone talking down to you like they know something that you don't know or should know? This better-than -- less-than type of posturing is demeaning and another ghoulish reflection of D-Con that arose from constantly having to justify our existence by proving we are worthy. This reaction always comes from lack of self-acceptance.

Isn't it strange how the word '*therapist*' actually spells *the rapist*? I am not suggesting that a psychiatrist, or psychologist, are not a viable avenue of self-awareness, nor am I suggesting that we do not have things to learn from one another. Rather, I am saying that once we develop friendships with our peers, we can have relationships that perform the function of a therapist because we begin to move away from needing confidentiality or needing to pay someone to receive us and keep secrets for us. Peerage is about exposing the secrets we keep from ourselves...the very secrets that eventually get buried in denial. Once these denials are witnessed by our consciousness, we can forgive ourselves, make reparations with others that were involved or harmed by our denial, and have much less baggage to keep track of.

The game of Pangasm is not about schooling each other on the finer points of living. It is a blessed sharing of innocent intimacy between equals.

So, here you have it, two people who are attracted to one another and going to the most intimate personal places without intercourse, without shame, without projections about the future and without any strings attached, except what is agreed upon up front. You can actually fly this magic carpet for hours and hours if you back away from the pressure of ignition by utilizing the techniques of self-expression, which are as simple as deep breathing, laughter, tears and possibly Vagarian expressions. And, yes, some of us like to wrestle, scream, curse, or make totally absurd noises. I have played this game with many men and have had unique experiences each and every time. There have been times that the game stalled, or never even got to square one! There have been times that we were able to stimulate the chemistry to such an extreme that we felt as if we had been dosed with an hallucinogenic drug, as we saw – each in our minds eye- a long line of colorful images of ancient peoples in ancient garb pass by us like a long line of ancestors revealing themselves; I have played from sun-down to sun-up and was able to feel as though I had a full nights sleep! I have developed great and lasting romantic relationships or established friendships that never approached a sexual relationship. But, I do not necessarily wish to create any preconceived ideas about the results that this opportunity provides. While at the same time, I wish to help those who play to understand how to relate to the unlimited potential for healing that this healing modality offers to unique individuals willing to create Heart Space with one another.

Sexual intercourse or oral sex is not the goal of the game. The goal is: intimate communication through honesty, the evolution of awareness of self, the expression of suppressed emotions leading to the exposure of old denial patterns, the development of the ability to help our body create the feel-good drugs of ecstatic eroticism, a deeper knowing and bond with a potential sexual partner, great exercise, deep breathing, tremendous entertainment that costs little to nothing, and heavy doses of sublime joy!

This form of intimacy gives ample amount of information to those who wish to seek sexual relations within the bonds of romantic love. Since sex is a very powerful action that produces substantial creative energy, as well as children, it should be handled with reverence and a sincere respect for potential dangers and potential miracles. For me,

The orientation of denial, (polarized emotional or intellectual) on the part of the participants, determines which direction Pangasm will go, how extreme denied emotion may be or not be, etc. Be prepared because denial is tricky and only gets healed through absolute honesty with self and the other. If you feel a need for secrecy, in any way, there is a strong indication that you are a prisoner of guilt and/or a prisoner of insecurity that is locked within the patterns of competition (better-than/less-than.) It is helpful to find a trusted friend and examine the voice of guilt with the intention of integrating the part of self that feels guilty. We are not trying to invalidate any part of ourselves, nor do we need to exorcise demons. We are trying to accept the lost and damaged parts of ourselves that were made separate through the beliefs we acquired from the Battle of the Sexes.

The person I seek out on a regular basis to mirror my intimate truth with is another woman. And since there is no sexual tension between us, we have been able to navigate for years in a healthy relationship, which is free and full of dignity. She is the one I run to for feedback about my life and my perspectives. Since I provide the same function for her, we are peers and true friends. We do not keep secrets for or from one another, because we do not harbor secrets as a rule…especially knowing that secrets indicate shame. Instead, we share our deepest selves and concerns in an atmosphere of honesty and self-acceptance. These types of complimentary relationships are indispensable to the healing process I am recommending and serve to help us become increasingly shameless and intimate. The game of Pangasm is designed to move us toward singing our own unique Heart Song as a means of getting to know our true self, instead of the presentation-self we were required to develop by the collective paradigm of our society.

This game creates a setting that is one of the most dynamic opportunities available to access the sub-conscious self without a therapist who could possibly imbed more beliefs into this very impressionable, highly un-evolved realm of our existence. We are truly delicate beings and we need to be gentle with ourselves in these times. Generally, the part of us that comes forward in these moments is under a lot of pressure from already having been rejected in the past. If this part of self meets with more shame, non-acceptance or ridicule, it could send it into a reversal that further damages self (a reversal is an energetic repulsion between the parts of self). Please know we are healing damaged and wounded parts of self that have been living in the hell of denied-darkness. So please handle these un-evolved parts of self with liberal amounts of Heart Space. Even though I call this a game, and, it is, I want to convey that it is most helpful to have a consciousness of BEING to be present that knows this experience is a "coming out of our closet" event. If the partners acknowledge this aspect of the game ahead of time and express mutual desire to handle each other with care, both of you will experience the power that Heart-Space brings by way of simple agreement and honest straightforwardness. It is through Pangasm that the art of evolutionary honesty can begin to reveal the magic that is our birthright. This opening to genuine intimacy is so fascinating and powerful that you may draw the same conclusion I did…that non-sexual *Pangasmic Heart Space* is the second best form of satisfaction. The best is, of course, great sex within Heart-Space!

Heart Space is that precious place that accepts self and the other as we are in this present moment…even if we are out of balance. It is the ability to accept one's current level of denial that will enable us to create a safe place to resolve heartlessness. Heart-Space can only be real if both parties are being honest. Heart-Space does not hold any form of non-violent communication outside of love, even if the communication hurts one or more of the participant's feelings. Having said that, it is more important to accept and evolve our self than it is to have acceptance from others. For the most part, getting acceptance from others, when we lack acceptance for self, is only an illusion of acceptance.

The word self-expression describes the action that is happening for our Light Body matrix while under the influence of the game of Pangasm, because we are expressing from our Light Body that which was stuck and unmoving. Once this magnetic ether begins to move, the way opens up for the reciprocity of evolution and involution to begin their special wave-particle dance of manifesting a divine Personality in a Body within time and space.

I try not to blame others for expressing imbalance because the expression of their imbalance is the pathway of establishing balance. Heart Space takes responsibility and is willing to tell the truth even if it makes us look, sound or act stupid, immature, heartless or negative. Negative emotions are simply barometers for ourselves to understand what we desire and what we do not like, as well as to inform us about dangerous levels of imbalance. So don't shoot the messenger just because the message is disturbing. There is a real disturbance present that needs to be expressed as a means of evolving true understanding and balance.

Non-penetrating sexual intimacy is an energetic vehicle for heartlessness to express itself within Heart-Space, thereby, healing the heartlessness instantaneously. All that is required is agreement, honesty and a generous dose of sexual attraction. I must repeat that the healing potential of this game does not work if both people are not experiencing reciprocal sexual attraction, any undercurrent of dishonesty will ruin the opportunity for genuine healing of the Heart. Sexual attraction is often used as a form of one-up-man-ship that invariably leaves less attractive people in the role of supplicating others for attention. Do yourself a favor and pay close attention to the voice that is planning any form of manipulation. Register your truth in order to integrate with the voice of hopelessness that is suggesting you will not get what you want unless you manipulate the other. This is the ever-present voice of abject hopelessness speaking and rather than giving in to self-hatred for our truth it is helpful to attempt to understand how the feeling part of us was forced into the predicament that rendered it as unmoving. This voice is not wrong... it just needs new information that will help it recognize that hopelessness is a deadly illusion.

Compassion for self and the other is a high use of our love for life, however, if we do not actually feel compassion, then it is time to express our lack of compassion so that love may fill the space that was stuck in hatred and/or cynicism. If you see yourself as ugly and unable to find someone who feels reciprocal attraction for you, then your body has received so much hatred that it has become like a magnet that is in repel mode with the hearts of others including its own self. People who feel this way about their body need to understand there is hatred involved in their relationship to Body, which is their unique relation to the Battle of the Sexes. Hatred for our own manifested body is giving the reflection of ugliness. This is a serious problem that is within the realm of healing, however, D-Con will not deliver any solution other than increasing levels of ugliness prior to death.

As a result of the universal Battle of the Sexes, we have mixed our electromagnetic ether with the other personalities that have helped us to co-create this hellish reality. Usually, when we are energetically entangled with others, it is because we have been co-creating experience together under the influence of D-Con and, therefore, made unholy agreements with our own friends and family about what is real and how to survive. These agreements keep us bound to patterns of imbalance and to those we co-created these misunderstandings. On earth, we have formed the matrix of the color spectrum as racial groups that represent the collective energetic matrix of our collective Light Body. We have been engaging in wars against our own kind as a means of attempting to control imbalance. Racial hatred is presenting itself today in stark detail. Our negative feelings toward other races represent our own forms of rejection for our own spectrum of being. Within each of us is the potential to maintain the color spectrum of ether that constitutes a human Light Body. Each color has a vital role in maintaining a full spectrum of frequency that is necessary to keep our physical form vital, youthful and free of pain. Therefore, having denied and not so denied forms of bigotry toward any aspect of self that is showing itself as bigotry toward other people or groups of people is yet more information regarding our unique Original Cause, and will give us specific insights about how to release the black magic web of self-rejection and denied emotion.

Our WORD is a powerful expression of our inner world. If another personality is haunting our inner world (we can't stop thinking about this person), there is a simple prayer that one can utilize to establish balance in their inner world. In this way, resolution will be freed up to come back around to help the misunderstanding get identified and evolve into a new agreement. I will say this prayer as if I were clearing with you because I am: "Anything I have that belongs to you, dear reader, I give back to you now. Anything you have that belongs to me, I call back to me now. In this place in us, between us and around us, I call the Light of Love to balance with the Liquid of Lovingness in the Heart of Creation." Caution: I give this clearing prayer with a simple warning that we are doing this for our own self, not to necessarily change the other that is involved. While out of balance, our judgment field will take form in the outer world and come forward to educate us about denial. Becoming obsessed with changing the other as a means of resolving any problems could only make things worse, because, as stated, our denial is forming these reflections; therefore, it is helpful to remember that we are altering our inner reality to create ever-greater levels of personal balance – instead of more effective ways to control the outer world. The 5th dimension is an accurate reflection of our inner world of the 4th dimension, once we establish personal balance people and situations will reflect this without us having to move outwardly. Having said this, if there is rejection, abuse and denial coming from a personality, we need to love self enough to move back from this person. Forcing ourselves to stay in relationships that are not evolving in a reciprocal manner is an indication that we are self-abusive, rather than a victim. At the risk of repeating myself ad-nauseum, I need to say that: *control is an illusion of the mind that believes changing the outer world will bring about inner peace.* Of course creating a lifestyle that is free from deprivation, over-control and violence, while also supportive of all parts of our self is a natural result of developing ever-greater levels of self-acceptance, and acquiring a healthy Will to live.

Over all, the game of Pangasm is a sexual encounter that does not produce any overt sexual interaction. It allows the two participants to energetically create the sexual drugs of ecstatic eroticism in order to learn what sexual essence is, how this moves, what affect it has on our sensory perceptions, and, most of all, help us locate and express the stuck and unmoving emotions that were originally denied in favor of being "good", "right", "proper", "safe", "righteous" or whatever it is that motivated us to be ashamed of our sexual birthright.

The rules of the game are important to uphold if the participants actually want to have therapeutic results. The Heart Space that this agreement provides is a great way to learn about the attributes of true intimacy among persons. Identifying our unique Original Cause around sexual dysfunction is a great avenue to locating our denied emotions and thoughts for our inspection and integration. Through integrating the denied parts of self, we become able to whole-heartedly express our desire as a way of manifesting it in the physical plane. Even if your all-consuming desire is for something as grand as World Peace, it is through aligning with what it is that we desire that we draw this to our self. This is considered magic by many, and it is the magic of personality we were all born with that enables us to create a reality that supports our Will to live, or a reality that sucks the life force from us... leading us to eventually look to death as a solution to the reality we created through various forms of continual self-rejection.

OVERVIEW OF CHAPTER SEVEN:

1. The most important rule for the game of Pangasm establishes that the genitals are a no-play-zone. Overt sex, such as intercourse or oral sex is ABSOLUTELY against the rules.

2. Physical violence is not an appropriate expression during the game. It is recommended that professional help be sought when physical violence is your reaction to sexual stimulation.

3. There must be reciprocal sexual attraction between the two players in order for the game to have a therapeutic affect.

4. Responding to the moment of ignition with sound and body movement is the pathway of purging our electromagnetic Light Body of rigid magnetic blocks that will also lead to releasing ancient thought-forms and guilt. In this way electromagnetic ether may begin to circulate our Light Body and establish Emotional Intelligence.

5. Creating a bond of Heartspace, through agreement among persons, is the pathway of establishing true intimacy between self and the other.

CHAPTER 8

EVOLVING PERFECTION

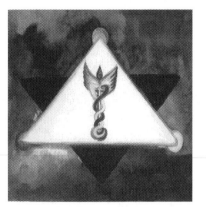

THE WILL TO LIVE

Here we are in a world at war, where violence seems endless as polarized factions of races, religions, governments and sexual partners wage war against the illusion of an adversary. As the disconnected fascist mind attempts to control the truth in order to present an image of balance, the obsession with being "right" has become the collective method of solving problems.

Personal Sovereignty is a form of anarchy that makes one his or her own master...unless one desires to over-ride the Will of another. Within the paradigm of Death Consciousness, intimidating form faithfully makes its appearance prior to death to give the participating personalities time to exercise their Free Will and act toward life or death. We find ourselves in such a moment this day globally as we examine the myriad forms in which we could prematurely experience our own death, as well as, witness the death of our loved ones. The emotions of terror that arise from this are the blessing of blessings that I beg you not to disown.

Fear is love that has not yet found a safe place to expand. Intimidating Form is caused by denied survival-terror and rage is the result of feeling powerless to affect the Intimidating Form that threatens to interrupt our existence. These emotions are the FOUNTAIN OF YOUTH that could extend our physical experience indefinitely if we were to develop true understandings about the role of human emotion in creating our reality.

Allowing the truth to rise up into our heart to speak about its unique position will move us toward aligning the denied fear, grief and self-doubt into a healthy presence that is in agreement with the heart's plan for radiant health. Denied negativity needs a safe place to vibrate the truth as a way of helping one to learn their own "original cause"...one's particular orientation to the Battle of the Sexes. When I allow the un-evolved voices to speak, these unaligned points of view integrate with my new understandings about the Laws of Nature. Tracking our own inner world with its incumbent factions of opposing voices can be overwhelming, particularly if drug addiction or alcohol is concerned. Rather than allowing addiction to take our personality to the brink of hell, it is much more helpful to face the source of our imbalance, rather than punish ourselves for suffering from imbalance by continuing to deny such. The Battle of the Sexes does not respect persons...it shreds them with regularity.

It is desirable to address our denial with the kind of openness and kindness that understands that terrible expressions of disturbance are not to blame for the fact that we have been living in the 3rd dimension ripping at one another's hearts as a solution!?! Clearing a magnetic field that has been stuck in a rigid un-reciprocal state for decades (and possibly lifetimes) is a tricky dilemma that is best done with others who are equally open about their own imbalance. How can I be open to that which is un-reciprocal without giving my energy to nothing, to that which receives nothing and offers nothing?

Every day that I bring more of myself into alignment with my conscious desire for perfect health, I repair my Light Body; I become better able to feel the truth about myself and others; I become more attuned to my heart and better able to create experiences I desire to have; and, I harbor less and less stress as a result. The function of the Human Will is vital to feeling our unique truth, however, in the current Human Condition our personal Will is supplanted by misunderstanding and leaving us like a ship without a rudder, floating on the whims of human factions that universally deny desire as a way of appearing virtuous. The paradoxical language of D-Con convinces a loving soul to deny negativity in the name of love and has created a culture of liars. This does not mean we are wrong, evil or bad, but simply suffering from a mass hypnosis based on an unfortunate misunderstanding about the nature of life. I am a recovering hypocrite and I place myself above no other.

Learning how to express my denied negativity and denied desire worked best if I were consistently to speak in "I" terms. If I choose to interact with people who don't tell me about themselves to the point that I begin to tell them about themselves, then I should move back from these people until such a time as they are ready to come out of hiding. Giving freely of myself while others keep their own inner world separate is a terrible reality to be stuck in. If you find yourself in these types of relationships, I suggest that you change your life by moving back from these people...no matter who they may be to you.

Lack of intimacy is not love, but is denial presenting itself as love. We will be able to feel whether this is happening once we connect to our own secretive places and activate our magnetic field by aligning with the Will to Live.

The intimidating form of the Melt Water event that is now happening on the Earth is creating violent weather and intensified volcanic eruptions and earthquakes. As a self-aware species, we have become numb to these frightening occurrences, just like the person who was raised in a war zone becomes accustomed to the constant threat of death from the outside. If you have the Will to live, you will more likely find a safe place to ride the Melt Water out. I recommend moving away from the edges of the Tectonic Plates where most of the violence will occur as the Earth moves to change the atmospheric status quo. Of course, the Sun and Earth have the ability to eliminate anyone at anytime, not just those who find themselves in an Earth-change catastrophe. Death is personal! It is either a conscious decision or a sub-conscious decision on the part of each individual and/or group that has a denied or not so denied *death-wish*.

When an individual or group has more of their essence locked in denial than is available to consciousness, then the Intimidating Form becomes the Grim Reaper. However, aligning our heart with life through emotional movement and judgment-release gives us ample life force to hold the 4-parts of personality together long enough to enable our dense flesh to co-ordinate the 5 elements into perfect health personified by a unique Heart-song.

We are not truly powerless to create a reality that we love, an existence that gives us security and peace. Aligning our heart with life will lead us to align with others that also desire life. Together we will have ample opportunity to express the denied survival-terror that has plagued us since the beginning of time and The Fall of Man. I refer to the *Fall of Man* to mean that mankind has devolved from highly sophisticated societies that had tremendous knowledge about astronomy and alchemy, then descended into darkness and estrangement to become the shabby remnants of this glorious birthright by constituting the age-old Battle of the Sexes complete with terrible reflections that accurately depict escalating depravity. Expressing the fear that died the last time we came to this Star-Gate will help relieve the anger many of us feel toward God and Goddess for subjecting us to such brutality. Honestly singing the denied terror, rage and grief Heart-Song of Truth will vibrate the Earth Plane open for a resolution and a time when we have the ability to access the truth of the ages through simply choosing to live as divine personalities who refuse to lie or override the Will of another.

During this Star-Gate, earth's vibratory frequency increases under the influence of the nearest Photon Belt of the Milky Way Light Plasma Matrix. The Photon Belts are the bands of light that we see as the great spiraling arms of our galaxy. These bands of light are energetic bands that lead into the center of the Milky Way. The Maya people called this Star-Gate event the *"Dark Path"* because on December 21, 2012 Helios aligns with the central sun of our galaxy (called "Alcyone" by some who interpret the Maya records) to expose the dark winding path that lies between two photon belts, leading directly to the center of our Galaxy to reveal a cluster of stars that resemble a Christmas tree. This potent symbol represents the sacred *TREE OF LIFE.*[5]

The Tree of Life in the center of our galaxy is a macrocosmic reality astronomically, as well as, a microcosmic presence in our own body. I relate to the glands at our crown (pineal and pituitary) and all the

---

5   We can have a more general discussion of galactic alignments in history if we consider that the solstice axis aligns with the galactic equator every half of a precession cycle. Likewise, the equinox axis aligns with the galactic equator every half of a precession cycle - approximately every 13,000 years. In terms of Mayan astronomy and mythology, the Dark Rift feature (which the Maya called the *Black Road*, the *Dark Path*) lies along the galactic equator in the place where the December solstice sun will be in 2012. (More precisely, the December solstice sun will reach the southern terminus of the Dark Rift, where it touches the ecliptic in Sagittarius.) Thus, in terms of Mayan mythology, we can also describe the Galactic Alignment of era-2012 as the alignment of the December solstice sun and the Dark Rift. This entire region is targeted by the symbolic CROSS, formed by the Milky Way and the ecliptic between Sagittarius and Scorpio. This Cross was also recognized by the Maya, and was called the Crossroads or Sacred Tree. This entire region is embraced by what astronomers call the *'nuclear bulge'* of the Galactic Center. As any amateur astronomer or naked eye star-gazer knows, this nuclear bulge is recognizable without the aid of radio telescopes. It is wider and brighter than other parts of the Milky Way. So, in a general sense we can also say that the alignment in 2012 is an alignment between the December solstice sun and the Galactic Center. However, since the nuclear bulge is quite large, this definition is not as precise as saying "the alignment of the December solstice sun with the Galactic equator", which occurs in the range 1990 - 2016. This is the alignment zone I refer to with the term *"era-2012."*

successive glands that travel down both sides of the human throat into the chest and all the way down to our groin as our biological Tree of Life because bio-spiritual balance comes from these glands when we are in alignment. When my personal Tree of Life sustains hormonal balance, I will be able to integrate with the heightened frequency of the Photon Belt that the Earth is moving through. By establishing and maintaining my own personal health first, I become a viable container for the liquid light of love, which freely comes from Providence, in such a way, that I am able to help others, if I so desire. What a miracle of creation our human body really is!

Our personal Tree of Life is also the mechanism that responds to our orgasmic chemistry, enabling us to combine with our partner's chemistry to pro-create our desired reality. Once a sexual pair agrees to create perfect health with their life force, it becomes possible to raise their vibratory frequency and lift the 5 elements out of the stagnation of death to match the rising frequency of our planet. This is the masterful simplicity of an **evolving perfection.**

Even without a lover, anyone who is choosing life and honesty may simply enjoy self-induced orgasm as a healing remedy free of charge. Yes, it is necessary to address the blocks and the false ideas as they arise, and, as well, it is also vital that we simply get on with the art of living.

As I awake from this nightmare of estrangement and predatory violence, I have become aware that my Heart's desire is not founded upon death as much as it is founded upon life. Therefore, I am able to forgive myself for selling my Soul to death as I give myself permission to reject death with all of my heart. In so doing, I am able to open space through a renewed vibratory frequency by taking responsibility and feeling the whole truth, which, in this example, is repulsion toward giving into physical death as a solution to living.

Denied rage that had become a rigid presence of hatred toward self, and/or the group, is a terrible vibratory frequency that comes from denying our negativity and results in hopelessness and/or grief taking over the decision-making process for the heartbroken personality.

Now that my space is no longer closing in on me from the pressure of denied rage/terror, I look out at my outer world and see the space closing in on society at large. Establishing balance within our inner world will naturally translate balance into the outer world while the supreme challenge is to maintain the Will to Live within a society that worships death. I am treated like a freak mostly, but my children are trying out my concepts about honesty, following one's heart and ceasing to project physical death as their future transformative event. They tell me on a regular basis how fortunate they feel to have been taught this while developing their personality versus finding out later. I do not wish to use my family as proof that this principle is tangible, but it is my superb privilege to report that each one of us is healthy, successful in our chosen occupation, and we are creating dynamic communication opportunities with our sexual partnerships. I am convinced that the paradigm of *Pangasm* is healthier than the one I was taught.

I am still, to this day, recovering from many decisions that I had made while under the influence of D-Con. As I integrate the denied disturbance of having adopted self-destructive thought-forms, I feel much lighter, and I have profound daily moments of ecstasy that are not necessarily connected to overt sexual orgasm or interplay. Sincerely, I have never felt better and my body is continuing to change in reflection for the better. Even so, the problems with aging that afflict all of us is a process, for me, of getting to know my physiology and designing a lifestyle that supports my body to the utmost. As I weed the garden of my mind, I find that much of the intimidating form I had fostered was the result of erroneous thinking that gave flight to emotional imbalance. This can become a **domino of devolution** that can consume our Will to live…a very slippery slope indeed!

Activating our individual Light Body supports our DNA strand to move toward operating on all 64 Codon levels. This vision is my self-fulfilling prophecy for my future. Until then, it is imperative to honor my denied-self by allowing it a safe place to come forward to integrate and balance with my conscious self. The split between the sub-conscious mind and the conscious mind mimics the current paradox of North and South failing to reciprocate. In this un-reciprocal environment, we seem to only access a minority of our brainpower and also seem to be suffering under a stunted and self-limiting paradigm that forces us to lose the Will to live...sooner than later.

Under the influence of D-Con, we have forever and a day been hooking up with other people who are polarized to positive/positive or negative/negative making it virtually impossible to approach a situation that would lead to recognizing our heart-mate. Free Will has determined our collective destiny and at this point in time, unfortunately, we are aligned with death more than life as a diverse group of sexual spirits.

As those who choose life begin to understand the Black Magic language of mortality, they will grow an ever-increasing appreciation of the *Language of Shamelessness* that this principle promotes. Something as simple as changing our language can, and will, transform our world and the children that are coming in after us. The populations of *Indigo Children* that have been shown to have more DNA Codon's activated than the larger populations are enjoying benefits such as immunity to disease and Extra Sensory Perception (ESP). These extraordinary souls have been coming in on the population of earth for a few generations, and it is by their very presence that the rest of us benefit. This extraordinary group is forming a new paradigm that makes sense to their heightened awareness. More than ever these highly evolved people need a sexual ethic that will enable them to change the character of the human condition as I humbly offer the Indigo children the *Principle of Pangasm* as an alternative to the current sexual ethic. Those of us who were not born with these evolved benefits need to open to the possibility that the presence of a whole class of souls, who apparently operate with more genetic cohesiveness, such as the Indigo Children, will up-step our own genetic makeup to acquire these blessings of superior bio-spiritual ability. For us, it is necessary to allow our Will to live to guide us in the ways of aligning with and accessing this possibility.

Understanding sacred geometry is an exquisite method of learning the parallels between the metaphysical and physical realm or the SACRED and PROFANE. Educating ourselves about our biology and our Light Body is a tremendous way to undo the propaganda of hopelessness regarding the health of our physical form. In this way, we can become empowered through self-awareness to tread the path of true freedom...freedom from debilitation, disease and estrangement.

It's like we have been these divine vehicles with tremendous capacity for free flight, but we misplaced the keys as we sit upon Gaia trapped in a flightless body and jealous of the birds.

We each have a Light Body that can begin to establish a viable resonance once we align the 4 parts of our Personality with life. Even our bones and teeth are mutable as all of our density can take its lead from our heart. It is the human heart combined with the spiritual consciousness of emotional intelligence that co-ordinates such a fantastic capacity as the freedom to live in a *State of Grace*. Literally, our Heart is the pilot, our Will is the motor, our Spirit holds present our uniquely mutable design and our Body is there with us always providing us with the orgasmic arms of love as we fly the magic carpet of erotic inspiration, a true state of SHAMELESSNESS grounded in the essence of self-love.

This is my game: I am grounded, temporarily, trying to remember who I am and where my partner is, all this time feeling like a stranger in a strange land. Now that I know that I have been estranged from my romantic twin, I understand why I have felt so very alone all this time, constantly losing the Will to live in an un-reciprocal state. As I express the truth of how this feels, nestled in the safety of my own bed, I come into contact with the wealth of essence that had left me because I had, in the past, firmly believed it was unrealistic or selfish to believe that I could have it my way...which is life everlasting within the ecstatic arms of my Heart-Mate as we eat from the fruit of the trees.

Please remember that somewhere between selfishness and selflessness is your own unique balance point. Likewise, somewhere between the mundane and the magic is your heart's special existence. Receiving our heart's desire is our birthright and not some obsession of our ego. Our ego is our personal identity, if we have been slandering and hating this part of our self because we blame it as the source of our discomfort, we are indeed in rejection of the finest gift ever received…OUR DIVINE PERSONALITY. As long as we operate with a paradigm that suggests that it is not possible, rational or virtuous to want what we desire most, we will persistently be at war with our self.

DESIRE IS THE ALCHEMY OF MAGIC.

I maintain an open heart about my future and know that my desire will manifest with time, because my Heart is in alignment about what I desire and staying true to my heart is how I determine my future. I choose to heal my matrix through self-acceptance, truth telling and emotional release (magnetic), as well as, judgment release (electrical). I choose to heal my body from the ravages of stress, which is pH imbalance. I find a watershed that I most resonate with and protect the source. And most of all, I give myself a break by not forcing myself to perform any task that is against my Will.

The primary problem for most of humanity is that they have supported an elite few to impose the paradigm of slavery upon the masses. This cycle will be broken with each day that more and more of us choose to align our hearts with life. This is the true nature of anarchy that allows diverse people, each with their own truth, to live together in balance without an over-lord. We do not need to give up our truth in order to conform to the fascist reality that D-Con fosters, nor should we allow the beautiful providential nature of anarchy to be classified as evil, dark, violent or wrong by an elite ruling class that is terrified of losing control over the masses. Moving outward violently to oppose this ruling class is simply a misunderstanding about our power. By resolving the Battle of the

Sexes within, rather than without, we will be contributing to the precepts of True Free Will and find self-love instead of hostility.

As an evolving perfection, I evolve my own truth as a learning process about how to live, rather than how to die *"gracefully"*.

The electromagnetic ether that completes our Light Body is magnetized to our unique heart. Even so, it is possible to steal ether from one another because we have been under the spell of a misunderstanding called Death Consciousness...perpetually denying our life force access to its own heart. When we deny our essence in this way, it is up for grabs. However, rest assured that our electromagnetic ether will cycle its way back around to our heart simply because it is magnetically bound to our heart. This revolutionary process helps the willing to find the stimulation necessary to open the Light Body channel and make it reciprocal...even if one does not play the game with others. It is entirely possible to address an un-reciprocal Light Body without help from others. Sometimes we find our selves to be very damaged and feeling unfit to mix with others. In this delicate position, learning how to satisfy your own sexual needs, as one moves emotion and casts off thought-forms, will restore ourselves from devolution and put us on the path of becoming an **evolving perfection, rather than a devolving introvert.**

Ideally, when two lovers align with creating life-everlasting through their orgasmic chemistry, they have created a sublime Heart Space capable of changing their form and that of the world at large, whether the pair are 'Soul-Mates' or not. In my opinion, it is not essential to know who our soul mate is at this time, but, it is more important to begin aligning the parts of self as a means of knowing self first and foremost. Overall, it is important to tell our truth to our sexual partner as a way of identifying whether or not we are truly compatible. Our twin will show up once we establish our own integrity. By making sure our inner-word is aligned with our outer word, we may consistently move in this direction.

You would be surprised at how rapid one's awareness expands when released from the pits of self-rejection. Feeling ashamed of emotional imbalance definitely contributes to maintaining the imbalance. Identifying the imbalance with a healthy dose of self-acceptance is the only pathway of resolving the problem. I do not want to be humiliated or the only one in the room exposing my un-evolved truth, which is why I created this game. In this way, the Principle can be understood and create a ground for the types of communication that are the hallmarks of Personal Sovereignty and intimacy between sexual pairs. By simply changing our language, the world will transform rapidly -- I kid you not!

Orgasm is a powerful form of prayer capable of ending violence and injustice rapidly. Once we agree to never over-ride the Will of others, we can also make agreements with our lover to ask our life force to work from a distance to help others or even to heal one or both of you. However, if we attempt to align with our lover to use our orgasmic essence to harm others, the essence will boomerang (go out from and come back to you) with an exponential force to establish justice. During the Star-Gate "Phase-shift", people who attempt to harm others will have nowhere to hide from this type of Black Magic... nor should they.

Sexual alignment within Heart-Space is a beautiful way to make love and to pray for what we desire to experience. As we move to do this with our lover, know that any denial that is in opposition to our conscious desire will reveal itself. In these challenging moments I try to remember that neither myself or my partner are to blame for imbalance. If you feel blaming rage toward your partner, it will be helpful to keep your words of emotional release and judgment identification within the 'I' range, rather than trying to tell your partner who they are or what they should do about the imbalance. If we concern ourselves with expressing our truth, we will free our partner to do the same while maintaining their own dignity. If our truth telling is not being reciprocated by our partner, it is important to move away from this person because allowing ourselves to be denied in this way is self-abuse not self love.

Our word is a powerful song that can be used to ask for what we want. Keeping that in mind, when we have denied our truth for a life-time much of what approaches us from the outer world will be reflections for us about our currently held denial. This is a tricky trap to free our selves from, but I am proof that even highly damaged individuals can recover from death. If this is your goal, it is important to know that when we become sexual with others, it is crucial that we honestly examine any shame that may be present. Keeping secrets from others is a good indication that there is shame. Orgasm in the presence of guilt is dangerous spiritually, as well as physically! I grew up in the generation of FREE LOVE and I am here to warn you that this idea is an IDEAL for society to move toward, but going past shame to have sexual freedom creates hell on earth. I do not mean to be derisive here, but I do know that the cyclical nature of the hellish reflection that modern media is now painfully revealing will not shift if guilt is able to continue shaping the collective paradigm.

Having sex with another person is a big commitment that needs to be discussed prior to the act of sex. Communication is essential to evolutionary relationships and it is vital to our wellbeing to reach consensual alignment with our would-be lover as to what sexual intercourse means for the relationship. By agreeing on what type of relationship we would like to take part in, as a result of joining sexually, we create a viable Heart Space that establishes an energetic sanctuary – a ground for intimacy to flourish. For me, I like to keep honesty as the only rule -- however, many people like to create limits upon sexual expression with others as a means of feeling safe. Overall, it is important to know what you want and to ask for it.

True peace in the Arms of Love is the great adventure of life in a body on earth as a sexual personality. Since we were created sexual beings, it only makes sense that the Will of Creation is in alignment with our indulging in our sexual nature; however, sexual shame leads many to make sub-conscious decisions about themselves that may lead them to project any number of punishments into their future because they feel guilty and expect punishment. It is normal to feel this way when we break with the laws of nature. It is also normal to feel this way when we break "norms" and "mores" (social laws). The problem with this is that the social laws are based on holding down our truth as a means of survival and as a means of presenting an image of balance that is attempting to be "appropriate"...instead of authentic. This anti-dynamic of life is an insidious form of self-doubt that is about to reach such a dense state of denial on earth that the backlash of this collective denial could reach a quantum mass of pressure as to unleash the FIRE AND DAMNATION that religionists keep warning us about.

Sex in the presence of guilt will generally bring forward that which is in a state of denial. When we unleash these hidden places to come forward for integration through the process of Pangasm, it is important to remember that the feelings of distress need to be accepted and expressed rather than exorcized as if this were not a part of us. Casting the distress of imbalance away from, instead of taking responsibility for, will only keep the cycle of denial and projection present. This is why it is helpful to be with others that are genuinely taking responsibility for their own imbalance.

If you are not ready for peace and forgiveness, there is nothing that you may do to remain on earth for the transition I speak of. It will become more and more difficult to gather essence for more war. For those who continue to choose the ways of war, the rapid increase in the earth's vibratory frequency will shatter the neuro-hormonal-chemical matrix of all those who over-ride the Will of another. The reason I can say this with such certainty is because the vibration of Love will not sustain that which is in fundamental electromagnetic rejection of itself intellectually, physically, emotionally or spiritually for any great length of time...particularly now, during this epochal Star-Gate which is ushering in humanity's Emotional Intelligence.

The resonant frequency of the Photon Belt is a tangible form of life force that is filling our world with the frequency of Love and Light. In the past, this light had been experienced as a hot and punishing light because our matrix had never been cohesive enough to hold itself together while under the influence of the paradigm of death. The violent arcing method of an un-reciprocal energy exchange has made the white light strike as if it were lightning because the alternating current of the magnetic field could not hold itself together well enough to establish a ground. In order for the white light to refract into the dense colors that constitute a full-spectrum Light Body, the heart has to maintain reciprocal exchange between the electric ether (North) and the magnetic ether (South) as a means of activating East and West, or the Heart Twins of Romantic Love, sometimes referred to as the "left or right brain". When our life force is circulating our matrix in its entirety, it maintains a viable resonant frequency that makes the flesh take on magical qualities, transforming Heartlessness into Heart Space and giving one a sense of peace and inspiration.

OVERVIEW OF CHAPTER EIGHT:

1. Personal Sovereignty is a form of anarchy that makes one their own master unless one desires to over-ride the Will of another or harm self or others.

2. Fear and anger are Love suffering from imbalance.

3. Gaia's Melt-Water event coincides with the 26,000-year Precession Cycle of the Constellation Orion -- marked by the alignment of Helios with the central sun of the Milky Way Galaxy heralding a New Age.

4. The Indigo Children (among others around the world) represent a new genetic class that have greater access to their DNA in ways that will help those of us who have preceded them to access more of our DNA and activate latent parts of our brain.

5. By clearing the thought-forms of death and moving denied emotion that is associated with this, we become the people we were meant to be...a personality that has chosen to speak the truth of their desire in a way that draws reciprocal intimacy and balance.

CHAPTER 9

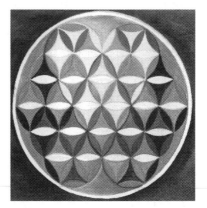

THE ENNEAD OF AGREEMENT

Agreement among persons creates *HEART SPACE*. When one is able to establish heart space between their own upper and lower worlds they will have the ability to design a life that pleases the heart, create a life filled with intimacy, agreement and sustainable balance. As witnessed by Dr. Emoto's study of water, the physical realm is highly responsive to consciousness. We did not truly believe this in the past because our own body had not responded to our conscious desire for perfect health. The reason Body has been so unresponsive in the past is because we have been split from our emotional body and effectually rendered heartless by our plan for death. In this respect, Body has been faithfully fulfilling its mandate as set forward by the self-concept of the personality, which is to create physical death as the future transformative event. We have been working at cross-purposes with the fundamental magic that life desires to manifest such as an evolving perfection that is like having our own Genii in a Bottle.

The world has been witness to World War over and over again! Today, our world is ramping up the pressure from our collective denial to the point of having a collapse, yet again, where a few survive to repopulate the earth, or we could participate in a collective revolution of human understanding capable of ending war and holding our societies together with heartfelt consent. Attempting to predict the future is a futile pastime...as in "Self-fulfilling Prophecies" put forward by Prophets who have given up on earthly ways, most likely because of their imagined glorious destiny that death would deliver! It is time to set forward prophecies of balance, peace, health and brotherhood, and time to imagine our fondest dreams while expressing the distress that had mired hope into cynical silence.

Prior to the Tahitian warlords appearance, Hawaiian tribes perfected the art of warfare within the context of *HO'OPONO'PONO*. This is the spiritual basis of the ancient (pre-contact) Hawaiian culture that can serve to set the stage for humanity to fight future wars within the spirit of non-violence. When different clans had controversy with one another, to the point of being motivated to go to war, they would gather in a neutral place to implement the rules and techniques of creating balance, that was known as HO'OPONO'PONO. Both armies would come in full war costume and, as well, all the tribal members of each camp would gather behind their perspective army. The warriors would line up in single file facing the opposing side and move in threatening ways screaming the cries of war, but they would not cross the line in the sand that kept them separate in their mass display of enraged warrior expressions from the other clan. Each side would carry on like this until they had exhausted their expressions of war. Even the villagers standing behind their warriors would hurl insults and accusations at the other tribe. After both sides had expressed until they no longer had the desire to, everyone would have a Luau (feast) with the families of both sides sharing a meal and music after the battle, thus restoring balance in a non-violent manner.

Every nation on earth could create such a gathering place at the borders with their neighboring nations for tensions to be aired as a means of keeping peace. I choose HO'OPONO'PONO and, please, I implore all the WOMEN OF THE WORLD to help me in supporting a new and non-violent means of warfare for the human race.

Today, war is posturing across the mainstream media reflecting the truth of our collective concept in the hope that we will recognize this pattern and evolve a new paradigm that no longer worships death and war as a solution to life. I ask Body to end this conflict by forming His sword into plow shears and putting His mighty efforts into feeding the poor. I assure you that this conflict is reaching a peak that has always crumbled the sandcastles of mankind. If you are praying for death and destruction as a means of setting things in order, then this is what you will receive on a personal level. If you are choosing life, the only thing you need do is clear your magnetic matrix of its death-charge, thereby, restoring personal balance.

Our Will is a magnificent presence of BEING if allowed to move freely. It will balance the negative vortex of darkness with the Light of Love so that "L" energy may flood our channel to fulfill the power of personal sovereignty. Our prayers for peace are not in vain just because the time variable has taken seemingly forever. Clearing our own personal Light Body is a potent way to change the outer world and honesty is the only method that will lead us into the sovereignty of personality that has the ability to evolve out of the violence of linear superstition. I forgive myself for having believed that speaking and behaving as I please causes me to lose control, to be rejected or get enslaved.

Control is an illusion of the mind that insists that the forces of nature are to be manipulated because the basic precept is that nature is intrinsically violent and inhospitable. This is not necessarily true. Through aligning the parts of my own personality with life, I have been able to direct the weather, plant trees and groundcover through prayer, and have found that the animal kingdom responds to balance in positive and seemingly magical ways. From what I can tell, animals can sense or see the colors of our Light Body and respond positively to a vibrant presence. Dogs especially respond to confusion and self-rejection with differing levels of aggression that I assume come from fearing personified un-mitigated duality.

Prayer that is uttered in a state of self-love has the power to transform our world as long as those who are offering the prayer are not over-riding the Will of others or harming self or others. These are the simple rules of the *Principle of Pangasm* that have the power to establish the true freedom of Personal Sovereignty which is a state of being that interacts with the outer world from a place of balance, emitting an invisible ether of the heart called "L" energy; the kind of energy that bonds hearts to one another and inspires communities to lift up the poor and dispirited souls within their ranks.

Until recently, the Will has been forced to stay silent about chronic imbalance and, as a result, when we finally take the pressure off from above and accept our truthful expression, the *Emotional-Body* will flip-flop around until it gathers itself together enough to hold centrifugal/centripetal center...Heart Space. This temporary disorientation will continually ease up on the pressure in our heart as we clear the matrix to become reciprocal. Every one that does this will have a unique process, so please, do not impose your path onto others because this is about personal sovereignty...not leadership. We will naturally stop our posturing and learn how to share ourselves, instead of supporting the ghoulish one-up-man-ship of survival terror, once we begin to feel safe exposing our genuine selves.

It is most important to remember that the negative polarity is not less desirable than the positive polarity. We would not be in a body if it were not for our negative polarity. Even so, the dense physical aspect of creation has been misunderstood and forced to perform death for the amusement of the gods that find themselves on Gaia in human form and trapped in the nightmare of their own insane holographic movie. Sadly enough, our persistence in relating to positive and negative as good and bad has demonized an entire spectrum of our nature. The negative spectrum loves the light and wants to live, yet, it has been forced out into the darkness of discrimination, essentially demonized by positive thinking that is in denial of chronic imbalance being called normal, love, karma, "God's Will for us", etc.

In the darkness of rejection, our denied electromagnetic ether loses the ability to move in its estranged relation to the light. Without the electric pole of itself, the magnetic vortex of the root loses vibratory frequency to the point that it begins to fall apart. This is when the space closes in on the vacuum of self to end the suffering of the personality that finds itself in an unsustainable position. In this place of desperation, the magnetic ether receives tremendous pressure to move into the heart for expressions of distress. If the truth of the problem is not identified and addressed, the magnetic vortex of the root either collapses in on itself or arcs out of the matrix in an attempt to bond with the electric field on the other side of the energetic gap in the Light Body's matrix. In physical terms, the equivalent of this Light Body gap is seen in the reflection of those who lose access to their nervous system after becoming paralyzed. Similarly, if electricity does not reach every part of our Light Body, the matrix loses vibratory frequency and loses function.

The invisible and silent war within the Dark Feminine polarity has gone unnoticed while the very tangible wars between the masculine forces of the Light Polarity have riveted our attention. The original cause of the split between the mother and daughter has gone largely unnoticed because it is in the feminine polarity and effectively veiled behind the mystery of darkness. In this case, darkness does not connote bad or evil, but is simply the negative polarity of the divine feminine realm identifiable as the archetypes of the mother and daughter. These archetypes of the feminine have been separate from the light of love on Gaia, seemingly forever, as sexual shame is passed down from one generation to another without fail. This highly volatile self-hatred continues to hold competition present as a power play that is protecting insecurity and shame as virtuous presence. The conversation that will come to the foreground, as a result of revealing the Battle of the Sexes, will cause great temporary upheaval and quite possibly eclipse the silliness of the masculine standoff around the world that is currently holding the intimidating form of ballistic missiles and weapons of mass destruction present.

ABRAHAMS WAR

Abraham and Sarah of Judea moved away from their families to create a new reality based on their newly forming ideas about Monotheism as being better than Paganism (the move from believing in many gods to believing in one God).

Once they were established, they began to forge a life for themselves in the wilderness, bonded by their love and their new concepts about God. After many years Sarah was apparently barren of child and Abraham was getting apprehensive because he was attempting to create a new tribe that would promote their new concepts. Sarah eventually lost hope about being able to produce children so she devised a plan: convincing Abraham to take a surrogate wife to bear him children, Sarah chose for Abraham a slave named *Haggar.*

Haggar bore Abraham a son and he was Ishmael. After his birth, it was discovered that Sarah, herself, was to bare a child at long last! And so it was that a baby boy named Issac was born to a grateful Sarah and Abraham.

After this miraculous blessing, Sarah became insecure about her child's position as second son to Abraham and convinced Abraham to send Haggar and Ishmael into the desert with no provisions. In this one action, Sarah was giving them a death sentence. Abraham struggled with this, but finally relented in Sarah's favor.

Haggar took her son into the desert and survived. Generations later, Ishmael's offspring went on to found the Islamic religion, just as Issac's offspring went on to eventually found Christianity from his parents Judaism.

Today, as a result of decision-making that was based on hopelessness and insecurity on the part of Sarah, the world is at war. As simplistic as this explanation sounds, it is seemingly small actions that set long-term events into motion for millennia!

The issues that were born with the sons of Abraham have not disappeared with time or denial and now, in the world today, the foundation of insecurity and slavery are reaching the entire spectrum of humanity as a monetary system that favors just a few; while, the masses are enslaved to archaic ideas that keep them in constant suffering and striving; with the women of the world paying a dear price as they watch their sons and daughters embroiled in an ancient and senseless ideological war.

Christianity (the colonialist) owns the technology of war in the North, while Islam holds the root that is instilled with rage about incessant slavery being waged in the name of God and heroism in the South (the root represented by Palestine and Persia). Judaism is wedged between the warring factions of Christianity and Islam and is holding the heart position that is attempting to conquer that which Judaism spawned through a secret Zionist agenda that pits Judaism against the sons of Abraham. Additionally, this heart position holds the strings of much of the worlds' media and is waging a heartless campaign as it is tasked, through further denial, to keep the enslaved root from rising up into the heart of Judea: Jerusalem. Prophecy claims that Jerusalem will be the place that the world will witness the resolution of this long-standing and brutal war.

The Mother/Daughter split in the feminine polarity is the split between the upper world (heaven) and the lower world (earth) in the magnetic polarity. This split exists within the heart of all women just as surely as the masculine split between the Father and the Son keeps the hearts of men embroiled in Un-mitigated Duality. Essentially, these magnetic repulsions between the parents and their children have kept humanity from evolving into its divine birthright. It is time for the son to come forward with his true position about his attempt to hold back the intimidating form that the father continually creates from the paradigm of death. Since the father (spirit) is perpetuating death, the son (body) loses faith in the father and secretly moves to undermine him in the same way the daughter undermines the mother for also being locked within the paradox of death consciousness. The shame that over-takes the son and daughter (heart: East and West), for energetically betraying the parents, eventually kills their own ability to remain honest about whom they had become as a result of D-Con. Compromised honesty in the presence of sexual shame is why the world is at war today... as in all days past!

Body shame is the silent stalker afraid to notice that it is indeed hopeless about physical ugliness and the loss of sexual vibration that comes from sex in the presence of chronic body shame combined with projecting death as the inevitable outcome of life. One of the symptoms of this, that acts to keep this unholy pattern present, is the ongoing rape of earth's children by so-called "loved ones". As a species, we are entering the Phase-shift of the Ages that will eliminate the presence of perpetrators, liars and energetic vampires. Even so, no matter what our personal orientation to this millennial problem has been, we are not wrong for having reacted to this by choosing to polarize to victim-hood or perpetrator. Having said that, we do need to take responsibility for this by replacing the blame and shame language of D-Con with our authentic truth, even if it is shame for being ugly and silently hating self within the abyss of estrangement. Welcome to the Human Condition!

The Mother/Daughter split presents itself among women as two extremes that are in rejection of one another, like two magnets that are similarly polarized positive/positive or negative/negative. This double charge keeps the two in a constant repel mode. One religious story that has been adopted by Christianity about the two Mary's is a reflection of this split: Judea's Mother Mary archetype has been revered as a saint for bringing Joshua Ben Joseph (Jesus of Nazareth) into the world...seemingly without sexual contact. The other Mary, Mary Magdalena, was the alleged lover of Jesus and was condemned as a whore by the dominant male Christian sect that established itself as the Catholic Church of Rome. These two icons from the past have established the reflection of the extreme positions that women are

Lori S. Dante

forced into as a result of D-Con: the saint (mother) and the whore (daughter) secretly battle over the power to influence the men among them, which is the core of this war between the mother and the daughter. Either way, this split is anti-sex and has contributed to humanity's denied self-hatred since the beginning of civilization.

Since sexual shame has not yet been resolved in the root (where women are culturally required to wear a veil to conceal themselves by a heartless theocracy), the mother and daughter have been estranged from one another in such a way that it has been impossible for them to work together to end the war between men. The failure of the feminine polarity to align enough to establish a non-violent status quo has ripped our world asunder with heartlessness disguising itself as love. Within the context of D-Con the feminine polarity is faced with limited options forcing a decision between two extremes of self. This archetypical pattern has been repeated for so very long that it is difficult to notice that sexual shame has formed the foundation of an illusory 3rd dimensional reality that gives no room for the human heart to flourish.

The polarized reflection of the mother/daughter split requires that the saint/mother must sacrifice herself to goodness (the greater good) while the daughter runs away from the mother to recreate the conflict with the men. This is the predominant pattern of the feminine war that has found relative obscurity in the polarity of darkness; thus, the demonization of the divine feminine has persistently supported the misunderstanding about the evil nature of the dark forces. No matter what forms of shame the mother suffered from in her sexual development, it is always projected upon the daughter once the daughter begins to emerge as a sexual being. In this way the perversion of generational sexual shame is passed along, without fail, to this very day.

As you study these familial splits, know that these primary patterns spawn numerable other patterns that help comprise the panoply of imbalance that everyone is calling life on earth. This analogy of archetypes is put forward to help us understand the two primary splits in the divine feminine that set a domino of misunderstanding into motion...not to further demonize these icons of the past. Even though East and West are at war today, as in all days past, it is entirely possible to shift this ancient pattern in a heartbeat by aligning our heart with the *Principle of Pangasm* and living according to our heart's desire, rather than designing our life to avoid the inevitable intimidating form that is actually a symptom of having adopted death as our future transformative event.

As we identify the predominant splits between North and South in regard to our unique personality, we will begin to notice the reactionary splits between East and West as a means of navigating the 'remembering' process of emotional clearing and judgment release. *Pangasm* is designed to help all who play it to eliminate the crippling effects of denied sexual shame and the stress of survival-terror by means of simple agreement called Heart-space. As we heal the splits in our own channel, the others in our family will naturally share this conversation with us in a way that will lead to ever-greater levels of intimacy and understanding. However, nothing will change if honesty is not present.

The earth change event of a global Melt-Water is the atmospheric shift of the ages as seen on the face of Gaia. The new climatic atmosphere that emerges from this event is determined by the extent that Gaia persists in Her cycle of Magnetic Minimum and Helios persists in His cycle of Solar Maximum, etc. The last time that the universal portals opened to put the spotlight of universal intelligence upon our remote planet, war was the name of the game and, as a result, our civilizations were wiped out by violent earth-changing events. Now, as we approach the scene of the crime we are completing another 26,000-year orbit around the central star of our galaxy. Here we are given another opportunity to remember our individual contribution to our own heartlessness and the carnage of our past. In so doing, we will be able to gather all of our faculties to be present for making new agreements that support true Free Will and the body that makes it all possible.

During this Star-gate event, the astronomical portals open from top to bottom (North and South) and left to right (East to West). As with the microcosm of the individual, so goes the macrocosm of the collective. In other words, it is imperative that the willing participants have a reciprocal Light Body or their results maybe less than desirable. In this moment of decision, I wish to emphasize the importance of personal integrity as a means of enjoying the benefits of an ensuing group alignment. This period of escalating frequency shift is applying increasing pressure upon all those personalities who are not energetically reciprocal in their own personal matrix of electromagnetic exchange. Reciprocity is essential if one wishes to enter the 4th dimension from the linear realm of the 3rd dimension. These laws are not arbitrary or unfair because only sustainable personalities may enjoy the blessings of the 4th dimension. This is what the Taoists call the "*WuWei*."

According to the ancient Shamans of the Maya, we are currently (2011) experiencing the culmination and alignment between the forces and persons of the "*Five Underworlds*". These convergent forces that comprise the root of this universe, are preparing to rise into the Heart of this local Universe (the Milky Way). Only those persons that are energetically sustainable will be able to sustain their presence on the earth during this transition. Those who personally establish sustainable electromagnetic integrity will not only be able to stay present for this "*Epochal Dispensation*", but they will also be able to direct it to their liking in regard to their personal experience. This epochal birth of a new group agreement (paradigm) will be sustainable because it will be populated by souls that have made a clear and wholehearted decision to choose life personally and serve to help others see, through demonstration, the fruits of this choice.

Our galactic matrix of stars will attain Star-Gate alignment during the Solstice of 2012. According to Mayan scholars, who studied the Mayan astronomical records, this is a Zero-point moment of the Star-Gate event that actually began in the 1980's and lasts until 2017. This impressive astronomical event ushers in a "New World Order" to be born in the hearts of all men and women who have established the earth's new frequency in their own individual Light Body. This astronomical matrix of stars places our planet as the Southern axis gate (or portal) in our double helix Milky Way Galaxy that is a macrocosmic example of the human heart. In other words, the inhabitants of Gaia are residing in the crucible where the lower world passes up into the upper world. It is imperative that we align our heart with life in order to establish a viable and open passage for a veritable orgasm of cosmic energy, or continue to war among ourselves and bring the heavens down upon our heads, yet again! We have been here time and time again and, this time will only be different if we cease to speak the language of Death in regard to our future vision of life together on the earth.

As the cosmic cycles align, the macrocosm must find ground in order to replicate itself. When the crown is open to the desire of the root on a macrocosmic scale (Star-Gate), there needs to be a reciprocal channel for it to travel in order to prevent another explosion in the Heart of creation, such as the one that wiped all trace of our sophisticated civilizations out prior to modern times.

For those of us who are choosing life, our ability to allow the essence of this event to move through us freely will enable our body to survive the new frequency that is already beginning to rise. I am here, I am holding tight to my ground, loving the part of me that was so terrified that it prompted me to listen to its fearful message and move to a viable position on earth in regard to water access and the meager agricultural endeavors that would ensure my family's well-being. This type of personal responsibility has already paid untold dividends of peace and prosperity for my family and my heart.

The geomagnetic upheaval that we witness today on earth and between people is the balancing process that is happening within the collective emotional body of mankind and represents the preparation. Anyone who has been able to cloak the truth in the past will find it impossible to continue doing so during this "*Sorting of the Way's*". When we gather to receive this event in the name of Life Everlasting on Earth, it will cause the human family to emerge from the darkness of the birth canal as a planetary family among other planetary families that desire to live without war.

Within the cycles of evolution, life always replaces death because death is an illusion. As we settle into our chosen groups for this event, we will be surprised by the rapid turn of events that blesses our decision. As to how this will unfold for you? This is a mystery that only you will be able to solve as we all begin to individually and collectively exercise our Free Will. I will not predict your future because it is yours. As sovereign beings, we can predict our future by simply asking for what we want. By harboring trust that life is responsive to our desire and by invoking what it is we whole-heartedly desire, we will be using our power of choice as it was intended for a sovereign personality. The ability to create a balanced reality through an aligned word is much simpler and less painful than more war.

The human magnetic field is recognizable throughout the Universes as a point of personal sovereignty that is capable of producing a unique reality. The human technique of magnetically drawing that which we desire to us can be subverted to also draw our worst nightmares to us. However, since there was an ancient agreement that had subverted the knowledge of our personal and collective sovereignty, we have been like boats on a random sea of misunderstandings, repeating the seemingly endless cycles of denied life. Fortunately, there is enough time and space on Gaia for all of us who choose life to experience what we desire as long as it is not harming our self or others. In this way, the perfecting evolution of True Free Will can help us create divine balance which is a State of Grace called Anarchy.

As that which worships death passes from Gaia, we will all receive our own messages from our inner world and outer world about any denial that may still exist within. Accepting these disturbances as information designed to help us identify the parts of self that are still steeped in denial will become easier and easier for us to identify. And, therefore, express the un-evolved truth into the light of awareness for re-negotiation and integration. This process is made dynamic by the interaction with others who are choosing life also. If we force self to continually stay present with those that are in denial of life, we could become seriously disoriented to the point of losing the Will to Live. The game of *Pangasm* will give us ample opportunity to commune with other like-hearted Souls as we make agreements to open to the opportunities that life naturally presents...once we stop planning our death.

When much of humanity shares religious prophecies about a collective death, it becomes apparent that D-Con is approaching a *Quantum Mass Death Wish*. We have been in this position before and, paradoxically, we chose to die and forget what we had created simply because it was too painful to take responsibility for such a terrible choice. When life makes its evolutionary cycle back to the Quantum Mass Awareness of this primordial moment of decision-making about life or death, the past, present and future begins to blur. The wonderful thing about humanity is that we have forever and a day found enough love in our hearts to accept the unacceptable and worship our "Gods" with the beatitudes of gratitude no matter how hellish devolution has been! However, hopelessness is a strange bedfellow and creates any number of ungrounded sophistries to convince us to sacrifice our hearts to injustice in the name of love.

I am here to testify that the dominant paradigm, which is firmly holding death present, has forced personality to stay present with death in the name of love. I know this may sound silly, even inane, but, choosing to hold death present during a climatic Star-Gate could be a suicidal move in the name of compassion for those that insist on choosing death. There are revolutionary options that do not require personal or group sacrifice, but they will not be recognized through the use of the language of death. The language of Shamelessness is a language oriented toward life that aligns with the concept of an *evolving perfection* rather than a disintegrating reality fraught with betrayal and devoid of intimacy.

As previously stated, the earth's vibratory frequency is rising rapidly, serving to challenge each and every nervous system that is NOT maintaining a reciprocal electromagnetic Light Body matrix. I have done my best to help you understand what your matrix is and how it was designed to operate. Now, the responsibility belongs to you to make a decision that aligns your heart with either life or death. Even though I tell you that death is an illusion, it is still powerful enough to hypnotize large groups of spirits into manifesting the illusion of death in the name of Free Will.

Pangasm is the sound our cells generate when we have the Will to go on living.

The Laws of Nature are conditioned by mercy, therefore, those personalities that wish to leave earth through death can and will emerge on another sentient planet that is willing to hold space for devolution as a means of evolution in the very same way earth was willing to hold space for us as we chose death, age after age, after age, after tireless age.[6]

In essence, those persons choosing life will be provided for, but Gaia has had enough of holding space for the persons who consciously choose death. Perpetually providing for those persons who reject life is a paradoxical responsibility that Gaia has faithfully delivered throughout our collective past; supporting each and every one of us to enjoy a choice of devolution or evolution at any given moment. Until now, we have collectively chosen evolution through the technique of death, at this time, earthlings are awakening to their birthright from billions of unique perspectives, and at this time, we can agree to alter the collective paradigm to be based on sustainable integrity, instead of group illusions that collapse the illusion, with regularity.

---

6   According to John Major Jenkins, precessional mysteries are disclosed by ancient Mayan, Inca, Egyptian, Babylonian and India's Vedic traditions. Ultimately, the Maya envisioned the alignment to occur in 2012 as a union of the Cosmica Mother – the Milky Way – with the First Father – the December Solstice Sun. Woven into Maya astronomy, mythology and cosmology is a profound understanding of Earth's evolving consciousness.

Gaia also has Free Will, which is her choice to make earth-changes in co-operation with Helios signaling an *Epochal Dispensation*, and is the macrocosmic choice of the Ages in regard to humanity -- a choice so macrocosmic that our race would never be able to deny it. The moment of decision that we face individually (as well as collectively) is similar to the opportunity of agreement that exists between the sun and earth. It will be the cosmic figures of Helios and Gaia that will respond to our collective prayer by producing what it is that we are projecting for our future. Of course, there are those that will survive any group death event to effectively repopulate the future generations. If so, it will be their offspring that survive the radiation and the genome transfigurations happening today as a result of earth's magnetic field descending to Magnetic Minimum (shields down).

In the future, self-aware generations who relate to the conscious and responsive nature of the earth and sun will determine the state of our race. In this moment, we all have a stake in the decisions that will determine the future state of our race and the environment that supports us. As we develop ever-greater means of communication, we also develop the means to make revolutionary agreements that will transform the world, as we know it; because, Free Will is supported by the macrocosmic realm as much as it is supported by the microcosmic realm. As unpleasant as war is, it is an adequate description of the death throws that rejecting life feels like. Feeling into our unique truth and being honest to the best of one's ability is the only technique that *Pangasm* advocates in order to remain present for the peace that comes from creating balance on the earth.

The Will to Live is a Force of Nature.

Our heart beats the rhythm of continuity helping 72 trillion cells stay in alignment with the master organ that integrates Heaven and Earth...that of our unique heart. Hang on tight to your manifest form as this war sweeps across the face of Gaia under the watchful gaze of Helios. As you navigate the confusion about what is real and what is an illusion, remember that your truth is real for you. It is difficult to experience our true desire if we are in rejection of our current un-evolved truth and in rejection of our birthright to live in peace. Believing we are powerless in regard to our personal sovereignty leaves us vulnerable to those who are willing to steal essence from us. *Essence theft is only possible because an individual is in rejection of said essence.*

Contrary to popular opinion, it is much easier to take responsibility for our reality than it is to turn our sovereignty over to those who we believe do have the power to control reality. Religion is an organized consensus about how to live and die, and government is the offshoot of religion that attempts to hold the balance-point for the organized group. Religion and government are able to control the group through discipline only because the individuals have forfeited personal sovereignty. These group agreements created by religion and government are only a temporary illusion of balance propagated by the linear group misunderstandings about the Laws of Nature. True and sustainable levels of integrity occur when every participant is complying from a place of desire, instead of a place of compulsion. Unfortunately, since we still dwell within the illusion of the 3rd dimension, we have not yet attained this vital awareness, which explains why our governments and religions tend to eventually descend into the pits of fascism, and why the United States calls itself a "Free Society" when the truth is that it is a Police State that imprisons more per-capita than other societies!

Self-control is a fallacy that is promoted by those that wish to create a presentation of balance, rather than express the truth of imbalance that would challenge the dominant-paradigm/status-quo. We are not wrong for trying to control our emotional truth, because within the paradigm of death it is not possible to expand without collapsing, so we have forever and a day played with time in order to prolong the death sentence we have whole-heartedly adopted as a self-fulfilling-personal-prophecy. This persistent pattern has led us to believe that this is normal reality or, in other words, God's Will for us.

The love that the Mother and Father of Everything has for creation is willing to stand by until misunderstanding has its day in court as a means of evolving a pattern of sustainable evolution through life-affirming Free Will. If we, as individuals, continue to put on the presentation of love and acceptance before this is actually our truth, we will lose the ability to stay present for our unique truth. Today, in the spirit of evolution, it is time to create a safe place for heartlessness to air its dirty laundry!

Love does not compel us to sacrifice our personal point of view for any reason unless we are attempting to harm others. The only reason sacrifice for the good of the group is practiced is because we have agreed that sacrifice is loving and essential and we believe this is the price of belonging to the group. The *Principle of Pangasm* does not advocate sacrifice as a means of creating sustainable balance. When a "loving" group does not allow personal expressions of imbalance to be heard because of irrational ideas about these expressions as being "unloving," then the group loses the capacity to identify the imbalance. If, imbalance is denied by the group further, then the group loses its connection to the truth only to devolve into an illusion that is fostered by the group's dysfunctional agreement-field.

The attempt to control the magnetic realm is a serious misunderstanding that will lead one into becoming a monster of fascism. Learning how to live with a magnetic field that is free to move is an art-form of self-acceptance that will create sustainable balance. After having suppressed authentic expressions in the past, the human *Will* can, and will, become erratic once the pressure from the intellect is lifted. After an initial balancing process, (that may seem extreme to many) the emotional part of us will find a comfortable center that is grounded in truth. So, do not make the mistake of judging the balancing process as all there is to the methods proposed by the *Principle of Pangasm*. Balance does not just occur out of an unmoving field because one intellectually wants it to -- it must first be allowed to express the disturbance of denied emotions that were held down in a state of sub-conscious silence within the clinch of death.

The process of getting a stuck magnetic vortex to move can be like a spinning top that is losing momentum in ever widening and lopsided spins --activating this vehicle is a reverse of that motion. Once the magnetic vortex of the root begins to move again then does the electromagnetic vehicle begin to balance out into a reciprocal perpetual motion that sustains vibration and motion. The oppressed and unmoving emotional body must be given a safe place to flip-flop from one extreme to another as a means of finding centrifugal center. This is the reverse of what occurred to stifle the emotional body into an unmoving place. Many of us will not enjoy this process because we have been indoctrinated to believe that having negative emotions means that we are a negative person. However, if we can create heart-space with other similarly afflicted Souls, we will not suffer in a vacuum of shame about our common experience of recovering from the perpetual imbalance of D-Con. The more we allow this type of freedom of expression, the more we will experience ever-greater degrees of reciprocity and health arising from being reciprocal. This transformation usually happens first within our inner world and, then, our outer world will respond with ever-greater levels of freedom and balance.

Some will prefer to be schooled by the outer world as a way of establishing inner balance, but I prefer to look at the reflections of the outer world as a way of identifying the denial that I still harbor. This way I am able to create balance within my inner plane of awareness without all the humiliation that feels like suffering.

True ANARCHY, in a State of Grace, does not require force in order to maintain peace. Many Westerners live in a police state even as they call themselves free however, fascism is the only result if we collectively believe in controlling the populace... no matter how representative our government may seem. Therefore, our good intentions about liberty and the 'American Way' are only empty illusions of Free Will, if we do not also extend this blessing to all of the citizenry. The United States is poised to demonstrate to the world what a shabby illusion of freedom that group denial is capable of as one out of every 75 US citizens is in jail today and our electoral process has been stolen by a corporate oligarchy. Take care America because the foundation of your greatness already has one foot in the grave. Having said that, the goal of creating a society that supports "*Liberty and Justice for All*" is the all-consuming desire of people the world over. Now that we are connected through technological means, we have the ability to study these connections to see the pattern of this current universal paradigm of death. Now that we have the scientific means to see that biological life is responsive to personality, we can begin to understand the innate loving nature of Providence and begin to accept our birthright.

Where there is a Will there is a way.

Knowing about the responsive nature of Providence, I now realize that the LAWS OF NATURE are responding to our paradigm by manifesting violent weather, violent earth-changes and a predatory animal kingdom that re-enforces the ideas that hold our collective paradigm present in a rigid state. By sharing the good news about the blessings of Providence we expand the possibilities and opportunities that previously were nowhere in sight. To accept our divine nature as sentient Personalities who can conduct nature to be supportive and shape-shift our physical vessel to reflect our energetic reciprocity is an action of self-love; an action that creates electromagnetic harmony that bonds individuals and groups through desire rather than compulsion.

It is not wild abandon that I am calling for when I sound this alarm about the ramifications of denying our desire. It is a siren to alert the lonely and downtrodden masses to the open hand of Creation, so that strife and sacrifice become tales of old that give way to creativity and camaraderie.

As alignment with life begins to transform our hearts in a way that heals our collective body, we will rightfully relate to the water in our body and the water everywhere with ever-greater levels of trust and intimacy. In this new environment, we will have a feast from the fruit of the trees and celebrate the divine inner-marriage between heaven and earth in our heart of hearts. It is my sincere desire that we

Lori S. Dante

all participate in claiming our divine birthright by singing a sublime heart-song as we move to the rhythm of Pangasm…the cosmic dance of sexual beings whom choose to create peace and balance on the earth, and under the watchful gaze of a benevolent sun.

MAHALO FOR YOUR ALOHA

OVERVIEW OF CHAPTER NINE:

1. Pangasm is the sound our cells generate when we have the Will to go on living.

2. Religion and Government reflect the various points of view of the dominant paradigm, serving to hold rigid ideas present that are based on conformity to institutionalized imbalance rather than Personal Sovereignty.

3. The Mother/Daughter Split is held present by projecting sexual shame down through the ages as a result of an unfortunate misunderstanding about the nature of Personal Sovereignty and the role of emotion and orgasm in creating our reality.

4. The Will to Live is a Force of Nature.

5. **DESIRE IS THE ALCHEMY OF MAGIC.**

Glossary of Terms

Battle of the Sexes: is when a human Light Body polarizes into warring factions that cease to reciprocate electromagnetic ether. In the case of romantic interplay, it is a situation in which two people want to do different things, but do them together.

Channel: the central channel of a human Light Body matrix from the root to the crown (North and South).

Chi: the Chinese term used to describe electromagnetic ether.

Crown: the upper-most point of a human Light Body located in or near the Pineal Gland at the top of our head.

Dark Path: During Star-gate - solstice 2012 - the spiraling arms of the Milky Way highlight a winding dark path that leads to the center of our galaxy to expose a star cluster that resembles a Christmas tree...as predicted by Mayan astronomy.

Death Consciousness/D-Con: the linear dominant paradigm of mankind that holds personality within the confines of the Third Dimension.

Electromagnetic Ether: silver electric ether (Chi) comes from the sun and its counterpart golden magnetic ether (Chi) that comes from the earth. These two aspects of the element of Ether should be able to exchange properties in our heart...the citadel of exchange for electromagnetic Ether.

Elements: Earth, Fire, Water, Ether, Air: the Five Elements of dense physical reality.

Emotional Body: The magnetic draw that moves magnetic ether to the center of our being -- our heart.

Epochal Dispensation: the transition between the past "Age" and the "New Age".

Free Will: human prerogative to choose a unique personal experience and project choices into their future.

Gaia: the name for earth as spoken in Lemuria.

Heartlessness: Death Consciousness separates the root from the crown in the human light body causing the center (heart) to collapse upon itself.

Heart-space: The special environment that is created by the Pro-Life agreement between two personalities.

Heart-song: our word.

Helios: the name for the sun as spoken in ancient Greece.

Human Condition: the collective idea made material by the global family of humanity.

Inner World: the inner sanctum for the parts of self or the 4 parts of personality.

Intimidating Form: the threat of loss, debilitation or death.

"L" Energy: A term coined by the Hawaiian heart surgeon, Dr. Paul Pearsall, describing the special electromagnetic properties of a human heart that is constructive, not destructive. This special energy can be passed between personalities that are not in the same location, and is the electromagnetic substance of Emotional Intelligence.

Life Force: electromagnetic ether conducted by the human Light Body.

Light Body: a full spectrum rainbow of electromagnetic ether that includes electric ether bonding with magnetic ether and extends out from our physical center as far as 55 feet.

Linear: a reality marked by a beginning and an ending as in birth and death.

Mayan Prophecy: a Meso-american civilization from North, Central and South America lasting from c. 2000 BC to 900 AD. The Maya priests were brilliant astronomers, observing and creating ways to predict the movement of celestial bodies and their relevance to their timeline, and those thousands of years into the future.

Matrix: there are many usages for this word...the usage of it in Pangasm refers to the electromagnetic network of a human Light Body.

Merkabah: a Hebrew term meaning "Chariot" and also an Egyptian phrase that indicates moving rays of light. Used here as a word to describe the nature of a Light Body as a super-human vehicle.

 Pangasm: a principle describing the nature of humanity's collective sexual energy and a game that two people can play as a technique to make the electric ether to reciprocate with the magnetic ether in order to create a functional, full-spectrum Light Body. The Principle of Pangasm creates a revolutionary language called "*the language of shamelessness*".

Polarity: the nature of electromagnetism is dual with positive sexing negative, as demonstrated by the yin/yang symbol.

Polarization: when the electric polarity separates from the magnetic polarity in a previously reciprocal electromagnetic bond. Also describing the societal and physiological ramifications that the affect of Death Consciousness has.

Pro-Life: This term does NOT refer to a US political movement to criminalize abortion. This term, as used in the Language of Pangasm, refers to the whole-hearted decision that a personality makes to align their mind, heart, emotions and body with the Will to live indefinitely. Note: following this book will be a book offering a concise treatise on Spiritual Birth control and methods for regenerating our form and enhancing sexual appeal.

Un-Mitigated Duality: the rigid patterns established in our electromagnetic exchange matrix by the dominant paradigm of Death Consciousness. The electric polarity reverses on itself while the magnetic polarity also reverses on itself to have two separate hemispheres of existence that are not enjoying a reciprocal and sustainable bond in our heart.

Bibliography

The Ancient Secret of the Flower of Life: volume 2

by, Drunvalo Melchizedek: Light Technology Publishing, 2000

The Bible: King James Version:

B & H Publishing Group

The Heart's Code

by Dr. Paul Pearsall: Bantam Dell

The Messages from Water

by Dr. Masaru Emoto: Hado

Sick and Tired: Reclaim Your Inner Terrain

by Dr. Peter Young: Woodland Publishing, 2000

Signs in the Sky: The Birth of a New Age

by Adrian Gilbert: A-R-E Press, 2000

The Urantia Book

An Anthology: The Urantia Foundation, 1955

The Right Use of Will

by Ceanne DeRohan : Four Winds Publishing, 1984

Mahalo for your interest in the Principle of Pangasm